Personal *and* Professional Growth *for Health Care Professionals*

DAVID J. TIPTON, PhD

Mylan School of Pharmacy
Duquesne University
Pittsburgh, PA

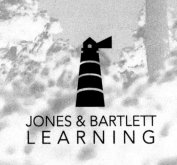

JONES & BARTLETT
LEARNING

World Headquarters
Jones & Bartlett Learning
5 Wall Street
Burlington, MA 01803
978-443-5000
info@jblearning.com
www.jblearning.com

Jones & Bartlett Learning books and products are available through most bookstores and online booksellers. To contact Jones & Bartlett Learning directly, call 800-832-0034, fax 978-443-8000, or visit our website, www.jblearning.com.

Substantial discounts on bulk quantities of Jones & Bartlett Learning publications are available to corporations, professional associations, and other qualified organizations. For details and specific discount information, contact the special sales department at Jones & Bartlett Learning via the above contact information or send an email to specialsales@jblearning.com.

Production Credits

Chief Executive Officer: Ty Field
Chief Product Officer: Eduardo Moura
Publisher: Cathy Esperti
Editorial Assistant: Jamie Dinh
Production Manager: Tina Chen
Marketing Manager: Grace Richards
VP, Manufacturing and Inventory Control: Therese Connell

Composition: Cenveo® Publisher Services
Cover Design: Michael O'Donnell
Rights & Media Research Coordinator: Jamey O'Quinn
Cover Image: © ChaiyonS021/Shutterstock
Printing and Binding: Edwards Brothers Malloy
Cover Printing: Edwards Brothers Malloy

Library of Congress Cataloging-in-Publication Data
ISBN 978-1-284-09621-7
Library of Congress Cataloging-in-Publication Data unavailable at time of printing.

6048

Printed in the United States of America
19   10 9 8 7 6 5 4

Contents

CHAPTER 3 | 49
Psychology of Professionalism

CHAPTER 4 | 69
The Dark Side

CHAPTER 5 | 95

Personality

CHAPTER 8 | 181

Millennials and Working Across Generations

CHAPTER 11 | 243
Professionalism at Work

CHAPTER 12 | 275
Professionalism as a Clinician

Preface

Your first professional obligation is to understand you, as you are the instrument that delivers the service.

THERE IS NOT A SINGLE healthcare student anywhere who does not believe he or she is going to be a competent, caring clinician and a consummate professional who is an asset to the organization he or she works for and the community he or she serves. To that end, professional schools and the students themselves devote extraordinary amounts of time and energy. Most of the time and energy is devoted to acquiring clinical expertise with small slices of time and energy devoted to professionalism. The forgotten variable in the transformation from novice to professional is the students themselves. Generally, the rigor of most professional programs crowds out time and energy for students to develop, reflect, and learn about themselves. Grades in biochemistry or clinical practice take precedence. This lack of personal development is a problem, because the student as a professional cannot be separated from the student as a human being. A student with an extraordinary sense of perfectionism will have difficulty coping with the rough and tumble of practice when things go wrong; the student who is excessively shy will never be able to take on a senior clinician who appears to be making a mistake; and the student out of touch with his or her emotional world may lash out when under stress. All the material and career success in the world will not diminish the discomfort of a practitioner who cannot get comfortable in his or her own skin or resolve the tension between personal, family, and professional obligations. Ultimately, this lack of resolution will impinge on clinical practice and will tarnish professional reputations. Not considering the individual as a variable in the professional development process is the equivalent of running a race on one leg. Linking personal growth and professionalism in a book has the potential to elevate both, because both are inseparable mirror reflections of one another. Bringing the individual into the equation also opens the door to consideration of the psychological processes that drive personal and professional growth.

Obligations to work, family, and school mandate that many students put their head down and then look up 4 to 6 years later when it is all over.

The economic pay-offs for this dedication are often substantial. However, this narrow focus in response to the rigors of the programs precludes self-reflection, personal growth, and enhanced self-awareness. As James Allen noted, "Men are anxious to improve their circumstances, but are unwilling to improve themselves; they therefore remain bound" (1992, p. 30). In an attempt to break this boundary, the book interweaves personal growth perspectives with discussions of professionalism.

Each chapter begins with vignettes that describe the personal and professional issues confronting four fictitious students. The students are as follows:

- Dana S. is an 18-year-old woman who seemingly has it all, a great family and a wonderful home. She is attractive and everyone considers her nice. She never lacks for a social life. High school was a breeze for her. She is abnormally reserved and hates being in the limelight or dealing with confrontation. If asked to talk to anyone but with her closest friends, she will blush. She really does not want to go to school; her real ambitions are to have a family. Although everything on the surface seems perfect, there are unspoken tensions within her family. She is considering becoming a nurse or medical technician.

- Ivan T. is a 24-year-old product of a broken home. His father was an abusive alcoholic who abandoned the family once Ivan confronted his father about the abuse. The result was a diminished economic circumstance for Ivan, his mother, and his sisters. Ivan had a chance at a basketball scholarship that vanished as the turmoil increased in his life during high school. For the past 6 years, Ivan has worked as an aide in a psychiatric hospital and moonlighted as a bartender on weekends. Ivan requested to work on the alcoholism unit of the hospital. His work in the hospital has sparked an interest in Ivan in becoming a psychiatric nurse.

- Niki M. is a 27-year-old woman. She is the daughter of an immigrant father who worked his way through college at night. She attended college on an athletic scholarship and majored in English. In her last semester in school, she fell in love with a charming man with little ambition. When she found herself pregnant, she abandoned her dreams of going to graduate school. Now that her son is entering kindergarten, Niki has to face the fact that her husband will never be the provider she wants. She has decided to return to school as a single, working mother. Given her athletic background, Niki thinks physical therapy will be a good match for her.

- Ryan P. is a 47-year-old telecommunications executive who has lost his job. He has two teenage daughters. One will be entering college next year. College was a struggle for Ryan as an undergraduate. Memorization and writing papers were a challenge for him. However, Ryan knows that he never wants to be "downsized" again. He is considering a nontraditional Doctor of Pharmacy program. He is worried about the cost, how he will fund his daughter's education, and whether he can actually finish such a rigorous program. Ryan is lured by the high salary and the job security of being a pharmacist.

The hope is that each student reading this text will be able to find aspects of the fictitious students' lives that resonate with their circumstances. Each vignette has been written to contain a personal issue and a professional issue confronting the student. Although I believe the personal and professional issues confronting each student are relatively apparent, particularly in light of the chapter topic they are linked to, the vignettes allow the students to project their feelings and beliefs. Variance in what each student sees should be expected and accommodated. There is no right answer as to what the vignettes should evoke. The vignettes serve as stimuli for classroom discussion and student reflection.

With most academic material, there is usually some attempt to relate the material to the "real world" via a case example. The reason to read these chapters and consider the ideas presented therein is that they should make life and practice easier and more effective. If they do not, then the time and effort are wasted. Clinical practice is a "full-contact" sport played by real people with issues and lives who are required to make clinical decisions while worried about their sick baby at home, how they will pay their taxes, and the rocky status of their personal relationships. A central premise of the book is that if you make better people, you will make better professionals. Learning to be a professional is not theoretical, a classroom exercise, or attained by memorizing some scribbles on a page; it is an inherently human activity. In making recommendations as to what the fictitious students should do, only completely nonperceptive students will not see some comparison to their life.

Most chapters are designed to be read in class and are written in a style that is concise and straightforward. The standard for inclusion of material is based on the student lament, "Is this going to be on the test?" Only in this case, the test is presumed not to be a pen-and-paper exercise, but the reality of practice. It is a best estimate of the minimum a student should know about these topics at this stage of his or her career. Think of the book and the course as a base coat of paint, preparing the surface for the colors and textures that practice and experience will add. This first coat is necessary; without it, much of what happens in practice will not adhere because it will be lost through lack of context, perspective, and reflection. Understanding how rigorous professional programs are, the book seeks to be efficient and judicious with the student's time and emotional energy for a topic that is a "side dish."

The approach to learning in the book is based on the following assumptions: (1) Students will see the value in this information and be self-directed learners characterized as curious, motivated, disciplined, methodical, reflective, self-aware, persistent, responsible, and self-sufficient. (2) Not all students learn in the same manner. For some students, personal and professional behaviors may be altered by association with a colleague; others will need to read something; and still others may need someone to talk to. (3) No two students will need to improve the same aspects of their personal and professional lives; thus a one-size-fits-all approach is not appropriate. (4) Finally, there is no express elevator to the pinnacle of professionalism. It requires commitment to a process of gradual improvement. Small wins in the pursuit of professionalism are the order of the day. These assumptions are put into play through the development of an individual personal learning plan.

The book is divided into 15 chapters. Chapters 1-4 present both a content and process model of professionalism and discuss personal and professional growth and the dark side of professionalism. Chapters 5-7 relate personality, emotional intelligence, and thinking and cognition to professionalism. Chapters 8-13 take an applied perspective to professionalism and discuss issues related to Millennials; creating impressions; professionalism as a student, at work, and as a clinician; and interprofessional relationships. Chapters 14 and 15 discuss the environment that students will practice in, specifically health care in America, and the legal and ethical context of practice.

A unique aspect of the book is the discussion on the psychology of professionalism. This is a treatment of the subject not found anywhere else. Professionalism is viewed as an ensemble of processes. Those processes are:

- Professional sensitivity—perception and interpretation of situations as requiring a professional response, what is possible, what is required, who will be affected, and how they will react.

- Professional judgment—which course of action is the most professional and what a professional should do in this circumstance.

- Professional motivation—what priority the individual assigns to professional obligations.

- Implementation—what skills, courage, and tacit knowledge are required to carry out the appropriate professional choice.

Each of these four aspects involves different kinds of cognitive–affective interactions with no cognition without emotions, no emotions without cognition, and no professional behavior distinct from the underlying cognition and affect.

In addition to the vignettes and the discussion of the psychology of professionalism, the chapters include the following pedagogical elements:

- Mind mapping is used as both a pre- and postassessment exercise of what the student thinks and believes about the specific topic of the chapter. An essential theme of the text is that what one believes or thinks about a topic is decisive in determining how they behave. This exercise is grounded in the ideas of schema theory and cognitive psychology.

- Each chapter concludes with an exercise that asks the student to enrich their understanding of the topic by discussing it with colleagues or practitioners and relating it to movies or TV programs they have seen or books or articles they have read and then discussing in class.

- Students using this book are treated as adults, meaning adults only learn what they want to learn and in a way that suits their learning style. To that end, self-directed learning is facilitated by the inclusion of a template for a personal learning plan about the topic.

- Questions are provided to structure comments and observations about each of the students in the vignettes. The objective is get students to understand that the topics under consideration are the everyday substance of what their lives will be like upon graduation.

- Students are asked to synthesize the chapter into a one-page executive summary and to be even more succinct and reduce the chapter topic to a two-sentence declaration of the ideas that will likely change their values, attitudes, and behaviors. The assumption is that within 6 months the students will remember very little of the course. The aspiration is that they will come away with 15 personally impactful ideas.

- Each chapter also includes numerous exercises and questions for discussion.

The objective with the text is to present the ideas in a clean, easily readable format that is respectful of both the faculty's and students' time and energies in a way that requires them to engage with the material. Passive learning or unexamined acceptance of the ideas in the chapter is not possible. Qualified instructors can receive helpful teaching tools including lecture outlines in PowerPoint format, an instructor's manual, and a test bank. To gain access to these valuable teaching materials, contact your Health Professions Account Specialist at *http:go.jblearning.com/findarep* or call 1-800-832-0034.

The topics discussed in the book are, in part, the substance of life and have been considered for ages. Although they may not be expressly declared, they include what it means to be good, how you make yourself happy, and what your obligations are to yourself and others. This is not material to be memorized, but tasted, felt, observed, and examined. Emerging from the course with 5 to 10 ideas with the potential to alter your personal and professional life is the objective. As you move through your program, ask the practitioners you encounter about these topics, about their lives, and about their practices. I submit that thoughtful practitioners will admit that the clinical side of things is easy and that the tension between personal and professional demands is the struggle. I know that this has been true in my life. This is a book I wish I had read as a student.

Reference

Allen, J. (1992). *As a Man Thinketh*. New York: Fall River Press.

Contributors

Robert Gallagher, PhD

Mylan School of Pharmacy

Duquesne University

Vincent Giannetti, PhD

Professor of Social and Administrative Pharmacy

Mylan School of Pharmacy

Duquesne University

Andrea R. Pfalzgraf, MPH, PhD

Mylan School of Pharmacy

Duquesne University

Reviewers

Cheryl L. DiLanzo, MS, RT(R)
Clinical Coordinator and Senior Faculty Member, Radiography Program
Montgomery County Community College

Suzanne Kelley, MEd, BSN, RN, RVT
Acting Program Director, Assistant Professor
The George Washington University Sonography Program

Jannett Lewis-Clark, OTD, MOT, OTR/L, CLT
Chair, Department of Allied Health
Tuskegee University

Hector L. Merced, MS, OTR/L
Program Manager Occupational Therapy Assistant
Cuyahoga Community College

J. Ryan Walther, MHA, RT(R), ARRT
School of Allied Health and Nursing
El Centro College

Wan-Ju Yen, PhD, RD
Indiana State University

About the Author

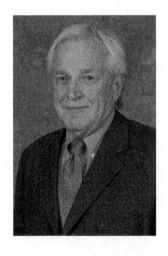

Dr. Tipton holds a bs in pharmacy, an MBA in marketing, and a PhD in management. Currently, he teaches in the management sequence at the Duquesne University School of Pharmacy, where he is an associate professor. Prior to returning to graduate school, Dr. Tipton was a partner and owner in a four-store pharmacy group.

Dr. Tipton has published in the *Journal of the American Pharmaceutical Association, Health Marketing Quarterly*, the *Journal of Pharmaceutical Marketing and Management*, and the *Journal of Social and Administrative Pharmacy* and has authored a book chapter on the Internet and marketing. He is Director of the Post Baccalaureate Weekend Doctor of Pharmacy Program at Duquesne University, the first such program in the United States. He is also Director of the Program in Health Care Supply Chain Management. This is a joint program with the Duquesne University School of Business.

Dr. Tipton is certified as a trainer in emotional intelligence. He completed a book entitled *Professionalism, Work, and Clinical Responsibility in Pharmacy* that uses emotional intelligence as framework. The book was published in March of 2013.

Dedication

To my sons, MATTHEW, SCOTT, and Joseph, and my grandchildren, Lola, Oliver, Scarlett, and Mona. Each of you is my favorite.

CHAPTER

1

Personal and Professional Growth in Health Care

Preassessment: Personal and Professional Growth in Health Care

Mind Mapping

*Consider the phrase displayed on the page. For this phrase, without thinking or editing, write down the ideas, concepts, examples, contradictions, and theories that come to mind. Do not array them in any systematic or orderly manner. Scatter them about the page. Now, draw lines between your additions, indicating that there is a relationship between the terms. If something causes something else, indicate this with an arrow. Relationships may be reciprocal, meaning both cause each other, requiring arrows at both ends. Indicate the strength of the relationships by darkening and thickening the lines; stronger relationships have darker and thicker lines. **Most important: There is no right answer. Do not compare with your classmates.** What you have is a mind map, your mental representation of these topics. Review to determine if anything has changed following this section.*

You: Ten Years

(What are your dreams for yourself?)

The Students

I

DANA S., AN 18-YEAR-OLD WOMAN, had a wonderful father. He was tall with dark hair, a great musician, a great storyteller, and the life of every party he went to. Men liked to be with him and women found him attractive. They always flirted with him. Her mother was nice, but not quite as warm. She had aspirations to move to the upper reaches of the social world in the small college town she grew up in. Dana knew that her mother was angered by her father's relative lack of ambition. Dana had a brother who was a natural musician and going through his rebellious stage. Dana was always described as nice; she never offended anyone and did not like confrontation, being in the limelight, or discussions about politics or world affairs. She blushed a lot. Dana was content in her own world. And it was a nice world. She lived on a lake, had a convertible to drive during high school, and had a date every weekend. She had a natural glowing complexion, luminous blue eyes, and looked terrific in her clothes. Her parents had sheltered her from all of life's turmoil.

Dana S. didn't know if she had been lucky or not. She was on the floor for her first early clinical exposure when the baby died. The baby had been born at 25 weeks. Even so, there was a high probability the baby would survive. All Dana saw was the attending physician talking to the mother and then this other-worldly shriek. The mother collapsed to the bed and started to sob. Later Dana found out that the pharmacy had made a mistake with the insulin calculations and had dosed the baby with 10 times the correct dose. The next day, Dana looked at the babies in the basinets and could hardly imagine that one died because someone made a mistake.

The episode threw Dana into a depressive state. No one in her family, or close to her, had died that she could remember. To Dana, death was an abstraction. It didn't feel like it did in the movies. Dana would never get the look of anguish on the mother's face out of her mind. Dana woke up last night in a sweat and could not go back to sleep. Dana didn't know if she could continue with the program. How would she survive if she had been the one who had made the mistake?

Both of Dana's parents were approaching their late 60s. She didn't know how she would survive if something happened to one of them. Also, Dana had never really considered that she herself was going to die.

II

Ivan T., a 24-year-old man, was always angry. He learned the behavior from his father, who was an alcoholic. When sober, his father was a great guy. They golfed together, played pick-up basketball, and reveled in the victories and suffered with the defeats of the local professional football team. When Ivan's father was drinking, it was a different story. He was a mean drunk, abusive and belligerent. His father often hit Ivan and his sisters. Several times, Ivan had seen bruises on his mother's face. The abuse only stopped when Ivan got bigger than his father and threatened to retaliate if he ever hit anyone again. Following this confrontation, Ivan's father disappeared from the family. Although the turmoil ceased, the money also stopped. His mother returned to work, and Ivan worked almost 40 hours a week in a convenience store during high school.

Ivan T. couldn't believe it. Things just kept piling up on him. He had always been glib. He could talk his way out of anything. Ivan had just met with the student standing committee to appeal the grade in the class he had failed. He did his best in the meeting to convey all the reasons why he had gotten the grade he did. Essentially, he tried to offer every excuse he could think of and had concluded with blaming the instructor for not doing his job. The committee told Ivan they would notify him by mail of their decision.

On top of this, Ivan's father had been diagnosed with liver cancer that had metastasized to his pancreas. The diagnosis was terminal, and Ivan's father had 2–3 months to live. To make the situation worse, Ivan's father had no insurance and no money. Ivan's father asked Ivan if he could stay with him in his apartment. Ivan knew he would have to help pay some of this father's expenses. Ivan's father asked him to use some of the money he still had available in his student loan account.

III

Niki M., a 27-year-old woman, was very smart. She went to an elite private college on a volleyball scholarship but would have been admitted on her academic merit alone. Everything came easily to Niki; she was driven and would do anything to make her parents proud. About to graduate with a degree in English, Niki had been accepted into an elite MBA program. What she really wanted to do was take a year off and travel, perhaps try and write a book. She loved to write. She knew this choice would greatly disappoint her parents.

Niki had just broken up with her latest boyfriend. When she thought about it, she could see the pattern in the men she chose. They all looked alike and tended to like having a good time and to not be very ambitious. However, being with them was so much fun. In fact, it was the only bright spot in her life. Although she loved her baby, she still needed adult companionship. The worst part regarding her last boyfriend is that she had loaned him over $1,000. It was money she did not really have.

Niki M. thought back over the last 6 months of the relationship. She had taken time she did not have to go to his apartment to help him straighten things up. She had done his laundry and had bought him some new shirts when the ones he wore began to look frayed. Also, all the men she was attracted to did not challenge her. She was always much smarter than they were and much more verbally acute. She could always get her way.

Because of her busy schedule Niki no longer could exercise or eat the kinds of food she wanted. Now, as she approached her 30s, she no longer had the toned body she had in college. Niki began to think that maybe she was going to have a hard time developing a permanent relationship, particularly with someone who was accomplished. Confident men who were accomplished frightened her. There was one, however, who had caught her attention. He was one of her professors, about 40 years old. The rumor around school was that he was leaving his wife. Niki looked forward to his class next semester.

IV

Ryan P. was a 47-year-old man with two daughters in high school. He still remembers the shock of being let go after 20 years in the telecommunications industry. He had worked himself up to a management position and took pleasure in his success and the recognition that he would be able to help his daughters with college. It took him 3 months to get over the loss of his job. Although his wife had been gently encouraging during that period, she was beginning to be more insistent that he make decisions regarding the future. It was time to start visiting colleges as his oldest daughter would be graduating this year from high school.

Ryan P. liked the long drive home after the weekend class. It was the only time in the week that he was alone and did not have anything to do. Sitting in class all day Saturday and Sunday was a struggle. Some classes seemed to fly by because they were engaging. Other classes were more tedious. During these classes, Ryan began muttering under his breath, making remarks about how boring the class was and how incompetent he found the instructor. Some of the new clinical faculty were only 27 years old. He didn't know if he resented them or was jealous. He thought, "If they worked for me, they would have to do things differently." When he left class today, he made sure the instructor heard his comments about how tedious the class was. Although he spoke in whispered tones to another student, he knew the instructor heard him. Ryan even tried to stare the instructor down. He remembered how effective this was in intimidating people at work.

As the scenery changed on the drive home, his thinking also changed. He thought back to his career in business. Although he had been promoted, he often had to wait an extra cycle for his promotion, and even though he rose in the corporation, his ascent was not meteoric. Ryan also reflected that some of his colleagues at his same level survived the cut. He was not sure how they did it.

✦ LEARNING OBJECTIVES

- Describe what personal growth means.
- Discuss the link between professionalism, professional growth, and personal growth.
- Describe what a personal learning plan is.
- Discuss the distinction between simple and easy.
- Discuss some insights on personal growth and change.
- Discuss Kolb's learning model.

✦ KEY TERMS

- Experiential learning
- Mindset

- Personal and professional growth
- Self-directed learning
- Wisdom

> " ... *personal growth precedes professional success.*"
> Wiersma 2011, p. 2

Mindsets

THE KEY TO PERSONAL AND professional growth is the belief you have about yourself and about the process, in other words, your **mindset**. Some have a fixed mindset, the belief that who they are is immutable and that aspiring to be more altruistic, or any of the professional dimensions, is pointless. In contrast, some have a growth mindset, the belief that who they are can be cultivated and improved and that, through effort, diligence, reflection, and self-directed learning, growth is possible.

Professionalism and Personal and Professional Growth

PROFESSIONAL DEVELOPMENT AND PROFESSIONAL GROWTH, in this text, are not the same. Professional development typically focuses on the technical aspect of becoming better at an occupational pursuit. Improved technical skills translate to meeting the professional demand for excellence. It is what school is about. Professional development, after graduation, is best handled via continuing education efforts. Professional development is a process considered in other venues.

Personal and professional growth are similar to one another in that both suggest change in a positive direction. "Personal growth is defined as any process by which individuals gain in awareness or understanding of themselves, and as a result, experience changes in their feelings, beliefs, attitudes, behaviours or views of themselves in a direction of improved effectiveness, accuracy, or health" (Wright et al. 2006, p. 738). Professionalism demands accountability, duty, honor, integrity, respect for others, and altruism. Professionalism requires the acquisition of the appropriate emotions, motivations (Glen 1998), theories about human nature, and

wisdom (an understanding of what is important). Professionalism requires the subtlety and tact to convey bad news, to entice a patient into compliance without resentment, to challenge colleagues without alienating them, to control certain emotions, to express certain emotions, to read a patient, and so on. Technical skills rendered without compassion, discernment, and judgment describes an occupation, not a profession. Rendering technical skills without compassion, discernment, and judgment diminishes quality and impacts clinical outcomes. Learning to drive a car requires not only knowing how to start the engine or shift gears, but also a situational and personal awareness of being behind the wheel that forestalls creating chaos on the highway. *Professionalism mandates personal growth as a precursor to professional growth.* For example, if a person has a negative bias toward a specific group of people, might not the professional demand to be empathic and altruistic be difficult? Or, if a person is extremely narcissistic, might not the professional demand to accept accountability for errors be difficult? A dulled pair of scissors will not cut if you sharpen only one blade. Professional development (technical skills) without personal growth (human skills) does not make a professional. *In short, you cannot separate the professional service from the individual who delivers it.*

In this text, professional growth is very specific and targeted. It is personal growth targeted at the values, attitudes, behaviors, and emotions that make an individual a professional, not the technical aspects. Specifically, professional growth is personal growth and change aimed at becoming more accountable, more altruistic, and more dutiful with greater integrity and honor and a greater respect for others. Understanding your personality type, cognitive frameworks, emotional world, and tendencies and expectations as a member of a certain generation is the first step to personal growth and thus professional growth.

Personal growth begins with the idea that each of us is on a continuum as a human being, with certain beliefs, emotions, behaviors, and traits that are more or less useful in fulfilling our professional obligations. Personal growth requires extracting from experience the appropriate lessons that enhance our professionalism. An interaction gone wrong with a senior practitioner is an opportunity for growth. A less than kind response to a patient's family that results in a complaint is an opportunity for growth. Each day in practice should provide the opportunity to grow in some way. In short, we equate professional growth with learning from experience.

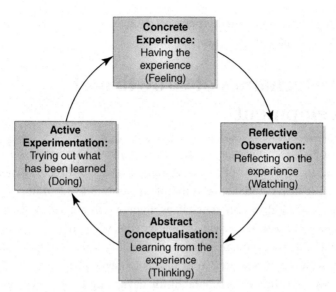

Figure 1-1   Kolb's cycle of experiential learning.

The dominant model for learning from experience is Kolb's **experiential learning** cycle as shown in Figure 1-1. It is a four-stage model of the following elements: concrete experience (CE), reflective observation (RO), abstract conceptualization (AC), and active experimentation (AE). This is how the model works. Something happens to us (CE) that we then reflect on (RO), causing us to change our mind (AC), which we then try out in a new situation (AE). Experiential learning and personal growth occur if, after a complaint is filed about us, we take the time to reflect on what happened and then adjust our thinking—for example, no longer thinking of people as insurance cases, but as patients. Thinking differently about the patients, we then test our new attitude in our next dealing with them. Doing this, we develop greater respect for patients and grow professionally.

The key to the process is taking the time to reflect on what has happened and then isolating and analyzing our underlying beliefs in that situation. If those beliefs impede our professional behavior, then professionalism requires those beliefs be either eliminated or modified. In other words, self-reflection leads us to change our minds. Self-reflection is an active and self-initiated attempt to ascribe meaning to events rather than just recounting events. From this recounting, inferences about the self are made. For some individuals, self-reflection may be relatively automatic; others may require a conscious effort. It is from this personal database that a personal and professional growth project emerges.

The Mechanics of Growth and Development

PERSONAL AND PROFESSIONAL GROWTH IS an exercise in self-science and can be thought of as a self-oriented and self-directed experiment. As such, it helps students to think of themselves as laboratory subjects. Imagine looking down on yourself, as if you are in a maze. What are your tendencies and patterns, when do they emerge, what are the circumstances, with whom do they emerge, what are you feeling and thinking, what is happening with your body, etc.? Your task is to develop an objective database that captures your modus operandi for navigating the world around you. This is a picture of where you are now. People learn about who they are by comparing themselves to others, by reflected appraisal (feedback from others), and self-reflection.

The mechanics for enhanced personal and professional growth center on developing a personal learning plan. The essence of a personal learning plan is that the student self-identifies that aspect of professionalism he or she wants to address. The student then identifies and implements unique activities and develops or acquires products and resources to address the particular issue. Next, the type of evidence that will be used to determine whether goals have been met are declared. Finally, a time line for completion is determined. Once the process has been completed, the student should reflect on the process and the outcome. A personal learning plan format is presented in the exercises at the end of the chapter.

A key consideration in developing these projects is that the aspect for personal and professional enhancement be as targeted as possible. Time and care must be spent in sharpening the focus. For a particular student, the general area may be linked to relationships with others. The student focuses on a specific relationship in a specific context; for example, the student's relationship with a parent over which college to attend and which program to select.

A personal learning plan is an exercise in self-directed learning. Self-directed learning is the only approach that will work with adults. Adult learners differ from younger students in the following ways (Taylor and Kroth 2009):

- **Self-concept:** As people mature, they move from being a dependent personality to being self-directed. As such, anything that is viewed as being forced on them will be resisted.
- **Experience:** As people mature, they have a backlog of experiences. These experiences are a resource for learning.
- **Readiness to learn:** As people mature, readiness to learn is a function of the perceived relevance of the topic.
- **Orientation to learn:** Adults learn those things that will help them solve a problem in real life.
- **Motivation to learn:** With maturity, internal motivation is the key to learning.
- **The need to know:** With maturity, people need to know why they need to know something.

Self-directed learners identify their own learning needs, determine their own learning objective, decide how to evaluate outcomes, identify and pursue learning resources and strategies, and evaluate the end product of learning (O'Shea 2003). "The ability to acquire skills in self directed learning may be the key link between undergraduate education, postgraduate training, and professional development" (Towle and Cottrell 1996, p. 359). "Nurses unable to direct their own learning will not have the skills necessary to meet the changes in modern health care" (O'Shea 2003, p. 62). Self-directed learning projects, done in school, model for the student a process for personal and professional growth after graduation, when the only enticement to learn is personal benefit.

Added Insights on Personal Growth and Change

THE FOLLOWING INSIGHTS ON PERSONAL growth and change provide added perspective on the process (Data from Tipton 2014, p. 5).

- To borrow from the book *The Lessons of Experience* on the development of managers, "The primary responsibility for effective management development resides in the managers themselves"

(McCall, Lombardo, and Morrison 1988, p. 10). The authors term this fact the "gut truth." The gut truth is that legitimate professional growth will be up to the student.

- Next is a change in mindset. If you do not think professionalism can be raised, then you see it as a fixed aspect of yourself as, for example, your height. If you think professionalism can be raised, then you see it as akin to increasing the size of a muscle; all you need to do is exercise.

- Goals come in two varieties. One goal is a performance goal; for example, to get the required grade to pass any formal course. A second and more powerful goal is a learning goal, to actually master the material and become a professional.

- No two students will need to grow in exactly the same way. Students will be deficient both in kind and degree of professional behavior. Thus, a one-size-fits-all approach to professional growth will not work. As near-adults, students will only learn what they want to learn. Under coercion, behavioral changes shown will quickly be extinguished. Sustainable personal change only endures if the individual wants it to. "Self-directed change is an intentional change in an aspect of who you are (i. e. the Real) or who you want to be (i. e. the Ideal) or both. **Self-directed learning** is self-directed change in which you are aware of the change and understand the process" (Boyatzis 2002, p. 20). Self-directed learners are characterized as curious, motivated, disciplined, methodical, reflective, self-aware, persistent, responsible, and self-sufficient with highly developed information seeking skills and critical thinking abilities (Litzinger, Wise, and Lee 2005).

- Not all students learn in the same manner. Some students' professional behavior may be altered by association with a colleague, others will need to read something, and others may need someone to talk to. How the learning occurs does not matter. What needs to be understood is that each student will vary in how they learn. Further, some students may get the "picture" almost overnight, whereas for some, it may take years. The point is that all students are different, and their learning styles and capacities vary.

- Mastering professionalism is painful. Nothing worthwhile is ever acquired without effort. Effort gives meaning to our lives. This task is just like acquiring clinical expertise; if it were easy, everybody and anybody could do it. Think of any skill you have acquired in your life, such as a sweet golf swing, learning to play an instrument, riding a bike, or understanding organic chemistry. All skills take practice. When asked the best way to get to Carnegie Hall, the musician replied, "Practice." Being a professional requires practice. You have to be willing to lean into the discomfort. "Learning to become an effective self-directed learner is probably the greatest intellectual and psychological challenge that an individual can face in a lifetime" (Dealtry 2004, p. 108).

- There is no express elevator to the pinnacle of professionalism. It requires commitment to a process of gradual improvement. Think of how a foreign language is mastered. Day after day, vocabulary, idioms, grammar, and the rules of syntax are acquired. Professionalism is similar. Gradually, the attitudes, values, and behaviors that constitute professionalism are recognized, understood, assimilated, and then woven into the pattern of a practice. No one loses 100 pounds in a day; people lose 1 pound 100 times over an extended period. Small wins in the pursuit of professionalism are the order of the day.
- No one is ever completely and consistently or perfectly professional. There is always something more to be learned. It is the recognition that the pursuit of professionalism is like an asymptote in algebra. An asymptote is a curve that approaches, but never touches, a straight line. On your last day of work, 40–50 years in the future, there will be some aspect of your professionalism that can be improved. Professionalism is not a dichotomous variable (either/or) but a continuous variable (more/less).

Simple Is Not Easy

Acquiring professional skills is hard. Acquiring personal and professional growth is even harder. It begins with self-reflection, a hard look in the mirror and the recognition of a deficiency. When deficiency is encountered, resistance emerges as individuals defend their ego and their image of themselves. The task is to avoid linking deficiency in a skill, attitude, or behavior with a generalized belief of deficiency as a human being.

On the surface, it sounds easy; be more empathetic, compassionate, accountable, patient, etc. The recommendations are straightforward and simple. For example, put yourself in others' shoes; do not let stress get to you; balance your personal and professional life. Think of the classic advice for weight loss: eat less and exercise more. Yet obesity rages. *Simple to understand does not mean easy to do.* If all your life you have been shy and introverted or seen the world through a dark haze of negativity and cynicism, moving to a more outgoing style or an optimistic view of the world will likely be somewhat of a struggle. Knowing you should not be afraid of strangers is much different than not being afraid of strangers.

The Goals of Personal and Professional Growth

PERSONAL AND PROFESSIONAL GROWTH REQUIRES a goal, an end point, a target to move toward. That goal is expertise in the fundamental aspects of a good life and a good practice. It is to be wise about both.

- Wisdom addresses important and difficult questions and strategies about the conduct and the meaning of life.
- Wisdom includes knowledge about the limits of knowledge and the uncertainties of the world.
- Wisdom represents a truly superior level of knowledge, judgment, and advice.
- Wisdom constitutes knowledge with extraordinary scope, depth, measure, and balance.
- Wisdom involves a perfect synergy of mind and character, that is, an orchestration of knowledge and virtues.
- Wisdom represents knowledge used for the good or well-being of oneself and that of others.
- Wisdom is easily recognized when manifested, although difficult to achieve and to specify.

People are not born experts. They are not born wise. They must mature and grow.

Writing about nursing, Glen (1998, p. 41) states that when practiced at the highest level, nursing is a profession that as an art "embraces a holistic conceptualization of competence…that does not refer to tangible nursing outcomes that conform to prespecified functional standards. Rather, it refers to the human values realized in social transactions between people." Personal and professional growth is a process of being more accountable for one's actions, more concerned about others' well-being, more dutiful and having more honor and integrity, more determination to excel, more respect for others, a greater sensitivity to professional situations, more motivation to act professionally, better judgment, and greater facility in implementing professional decisions. Personal and professional growth is a choice.

Conclusion

IN THIS CHAPTER, THE IDEA that making better, more self-aware people makes better professionals is introduced. Kolb's model of learning from experience is discussed as the theoretical underpinning of professional growth along with the idea that personal growth always precedes professional growth. The idea that the mechanics of personal and professional growth center on self-directed learning and the development of personal learning plans is presented. Observations and insights on growth are considered, and the idea of not confusing simple with easy is conveyed. Finally, the object of personal and professional growth as the development of wisdom, or the understanding of what is important in life, concludes the chapter.

What Do the Practitioners/Others Say?

FOR NEXT CLASS, BE PREPARED to discuss personal or professional growth based on any *one* of the following:

- A discussion with your colleagues, or others, on how they feel and what they know about personal or professional growth.
- An article on personal or professional growth, either from the research literature or any other source.
- A movie, television program, or YouTube video about personal or professional growth.
- A book on personal or professional growth (literary, historical, psychological, or any other source).

Personal Learning Plan: Personal and Professional Growth

USE THE FOLLOWING GUIDE TO develop a personal and professional growth project.

What prompted you to develop this plan?	
What is the general area for improvement?	
What is the specific issue for improvement?	
Why is this important to you?	
How do you generally act in these areas?	
What are your goals?	
What strategies are required?	
Who or what is necessary to meet your goals with this strategy?	
How will you measure success or failure with this effort?	
How will you reflect and capture the lesson from this effort that can be generalized to other circumstances?	

Identifying Topics for Personal and Professional Growth Projects

FOR SOME STUDENTS, DETERMINING AN area for personal or professional growth and developing the process may be difficult. Several methods for making this determination are presented below.

Identifying Gaps

On some dimension related to personal or professional growth, consider what your ideal self would be on this dimension. Now reflect on your behavior and/or performance in this area today. Is there a gap? If so, this is an area for growth.

Emotional Intelligence Framework

Chapter 5 discusses the idea of emotional intelligence in detail. Emotional intelligence is the ability to understand our emotions and those of other people and then craft a behavior appropriate to the context. Emotions are rich sources of information about ourselves and how we relate to the world. Emotional intelligence can be used as a platform for growth. Consider the following.

Strongest emotional reaction: Identify the strongest emotional reaction you have experienced during school, on rotations, or at work. Describe the context, the circumstances, the people involved, what you were feeling, how you behaved, and the outcome.

Hot buttons: What circumstances, activities, or people have caused you to lose your composure? The times that you "lost it" are areas for professional growth.

Fears: Think of the aspects of practice that frighten you.

The key assumption with this approach is that any area that elicits a strong emotional reaction or frightens you is a fertile area for exploration and improvement.

Appreciative Inquiry

Ask yourself what you are good at. This is a personal inquiry that seeks to honor the best in us. Identify what you do well, and then ask yourself how you can extend this behavior to another area. For example, how can I extend my personal confidence on the athletic field to confidence in making a presentation?

Learning History

Adult education assumes that as a person matures he or she has a backlog of experiences. These experiences are a resource for learning. The question is how to record these experiences and then access the relevant lessons. A personal learning history accomplishes this task. The process of writing a personal learning history is simple. Make two columns on a piece of paper. In the left-hand column, record a narrative, the story of what happened; for example, the story of your first clinical rotation. Write the story from your perspective. However, if you are aware of other players' points of view, incorporate these also. In the right-hand column, analyze what happened, looking for patterns and areas for improvement. The material in the right-hand column becomes the focus of your personal learning plan. Having someone else read your learning history will confirm the validity of your interpretation of events.

Critical Incident Reports

A critical incident report is a short narrative story of a specific event judged by the student to have significant importance in his or her professional development. A critical incident can be a learning experience, a challenging occurrence, a personally influential event, or something the student witnesses. In developing these reports, think of yourself as a "Monday morning quarterback" critiquing your performance for the past week. Capturing the incident is the first part of the process, but reflection on the meaning of these incidents is also required.

What Is Your Sentence?

In 1962, Clare Boothe Luce, one of the first women to serve in the U.S. Congress, offered some advice to President John F. Kennedy. "A great man," she told him, "is one sentence." Abraham Lincoln's sentence was: "He preserved the Union and freed the slaves." Franklin Roosevelt's was: "He lifted us out of a great depression and helped us win a world war."

What is your sentence? What do you wish it to be?

The Students: Personal and Professional Issues

BASED ON THE DESCRIPTION OF each student at the beginning of the chapter, what are the personal and professional issues (either immediately or in the future) confronting each student? Consider whether they are linked and, if so, how. Finally, what would you recommend to each student to resolve these issues?

Dana S.

Personal Issues

Professional Issues

Are They Linked? Will the Personal Issues Impact Professional Behavior?

Recommendations

Ivan T.

Personal Issues

Professional Issues

Are They Linked? Will the Personal Issues Impact Professional Behavior?

Recommendations

Niki M.

Personal Issue

Professional Issues

Are They Linked? Will the Personal Issues Impact Professional Behavior?

Recommendations

Ryan P.

Personal Issues

Professional Issues

Are They Linked? Will the Personal Issues Impact Professional Behavior?

Recommendations

Exercises

1. Look at the statements below and consider whether you mostly agree or disagree with them. Consider both personal traits and professional traits. What do your answers say about your belief in personal and professional growth? Discuss with your classmates

You are a certain kind of person, and there is not much you can do about it.

No matter what kind of person you are, you can always change substantially.

You can do things differently, but the important parts of who you are cannot really be changed.

You can always change basic things about the kind of person you are.

I look for opportunities to grow and change.

I am not really interested in analyzing my behavior.

It is important for me to evaluate the things I do.

I rarely spend time in self reflection.

2. Write a one-page executive summary of the chapter.
3. Review the mind map from the opening of the chapter. Would you change anything after reading the chapter?

What's Important to You in the Chapter?

WITH SEVERAL OF YOUR CLASSMATES, discuss the idea or ideas that are most likely to effect change in your values, attitudes, or behaviors. Be succinct. Write no more than two sentences.

References

Boyatzis, R. E. (2002). Unleashing the power of self-directed learning. In *Changing the Way We Manage Change: The Consultants Speak*. Ronald R. Sims, ed. Westport, CT: Quorum Books.

Dealtry, R. (2004). Professional practice: The savvy learner. *Journal of Workplace Learning*. 16, 101–109.

Glen, S. (1998). Emotional and motivational tendencies: The key to quality nursing care? *Nursing Ethics.* 5, 36–42.

Litzinger, T. A., Wise, J. C., and Lee S. H. (2005). Self-directed learning readiness among engineering undergraduate students. *Journal of Engineering Education.* 94 (2), 215–221.

McCall, Jr., M. W., Lombardo, M. M., and Morrison, A. M. (1988). *The Lessons of Experience.* Lexington, MA: Lexington Books.

O'Shea, E. (2003). Self-directed learning in nurse education: A review of the literature. *Issues and Innovation in Nursing Education.* 43 (1), 62–70.

Taylor, B., and Kroth, M. (2009). Andragogy's transition into the future: Meta-analysis of andragogy and its search for a measureable instrument. *Journal of Adult Education.* 38 (1), 1–11.

Tipton, D. J. (2014). *Professionalism, Work and Clinical Responsibility in Pharmacy.* Burlington, MA: Jones & Bartlett Learning.

Towle, A., and Cottrell, D. (1996). Self directed learning. *Archives of Disease in Childhood.* 74, 357–359.

Wiersma, B. (2011). *The Power of Professionalism.* Los Altos, CA: Ravel Media.

Wright, S. M., Levine, R. B., Beasley, B., Haidet, P., Gress, T. W., Caccamese, S., Brady, D., Marwaha, A., and Kern, D. E. (2006). Personal growth and its correlates during residency training. *Medical Education.* 40, 737–745.

Suggested Readings

Amabile, T. M., and Kramer, S. J. (2011). The power of small wins. *Harvard Business Review.* May, 71–80.

Branch, W. T. (2005). Use of critical incident reports in medical education. *Journal of General Internal Medicine.* 20, 1063–1067.

Challis, M. (2000). AMEE Medical education guide no. 19: Personal learning plans. *Medical Teacher.* 22 (3), 225–236.

Corey, G., and Core, M. S. (2010). *I Never Knew I Had a Choice: Explorations in Personal Growth.* Belmont, CA: Brooks/Cole/Cengage Learning.

Dweck, C. S. (2000). *Self-Theories.* New York, NY: Taylor and Francis Group.

Dweck, C. S. (2008). *Mindset.* New York, NY: Ballantine Books.

Fisher, M., King, J., and Tague, G. (2001). Development of a self-directed learning readiness scale for nursing education. *Nurse Education Today.* 21, 516–525.

Gardner, H. (2006). *Changing Minds.* Boston, MA: Harvard Business School Press.

Glasser, W. (1976). *Positive Addiction*. New York, NY: Harper and Row.

Glen, S. (1998). The key to quality nursing care: Towards a model of personal and professional development. *Nursing Ethics*. 5 (2), 95–102.

Hammond, S. A. (1998). *Appreciative Inquiry*. Bend, OR: Thin Book Publishing Co.

Hilliard, C. (2006). Using structured reflection on a critical incident to develop a professional portfolio. *Nursing Standard*. 21 (2), 35–40.

Irving, J. A., and Williams, D. I. (1999). Personal growth and personal development: Concepts clarified. *British Journal of Guidance and Counseling*. 27 (4), 517–526.

Kelm, J. B. (2005). *Appreciative Living*. Wake Forest, NC: Venet Publishers.

Kern, D. E., Wright, S. M., and Carrese, J. A. (2001). Personal growth in medical faculty: A qualitative study. *Western Journal of Medicine*. 175, 92–98.

Kleiner, A., and Roth, G. (1997). How to make experience your company's best teacher. *Harvard Business Review*. September–October, 172–177.

May, N., Becker, D., and Frankel, R., Haizlip, J., Harmon, R., Plews-Ogan, M., Schorling, J., Williams, A., and Whitney, D. (2011). *Appreciative Inquiry in Healthcare*. Brunswick, OH: Crown Custom Publishing.

Roberts, C., and Stark, P. (2008). Readiness for self-directed change in professional behaviors: Factorial validation of the Self-reflection and Insight scale. *Medical Education*. 42, 1054–1063.

Robitschek, C., Ashton, M. W., Spering, C. C., Geiger, N., Byers, D., Schotts, G. C., and Thoen, M. A. (2012). Development and psychometric evaluation of the personal growth initiative scale-II. *Journal of Counseling Psychology*. 59 (2), 274–287.

Sedikides, C., and Skowronski, J. J. (1995). On the sources of self-knowledge: The perceived primacy of self-reflection. *Journal of Social and Clinical Psychology*. 14 (3), 244–270.

Seligman, M. E. P. (2007). *What You Can Change ... and What You Can't*. New York, NY: Vintage Books.

Taylor, B., and Kroth, M. (2009). Andragogy's transition into the future: Meta-analysis of andragogy and its search for a measureable instrument. *Journal of Adult Education*. 38 (1), 1–11.

Wood, A. M., Linley, P. A., Maltby, J., Baliousis, M., and Joseph, S. (2008). The authentic personality: A theoretical and empirical conceptualization and the development of the authenticity scale. *Journal of Counseling Psychology*. 55 (3), 385–399.

CHAPTER

2

A Model of Professionalism

Preassessment: Professionalism

Mind Mapping

Consider the term displayed on the page. For this term, without thinking or editing, write down the ideas, concepts, examples, contradictions, and theories that come to mind. Do not array them in any systematic or orderly manner. Scatter them about the page. Now, draw lines between your additions, indicating that there is a relationship between the terms. If something causes something else, indicate this with an arrow. Relationships may be reciprocal, meaning both cause each other, requiring arrows at both ends. Indicate the strength of the relationships by darkening and thickening the lines; stronger relationships have darker and thicker lines. **Most important: There is no right answer. Do not compare with your classmates.** *What you have is a mind map, your mental representation of these topics. Review to determine if anything has changed following this section.*

Professionalism

The Students

I

DANA S. HAD NEVER BEEN so mad at her mother and sister. After much thought, research, and discussion with family, friends, and practitioners in the field, she had settled on applying to a professional degree program in nursing. Her first choice was a school in the center of a major metropolitan area about 200 miles from her home. Due to economic blight, the school was in a part of the city that was less than attractive and, at times, if caution was not used, dangerous. Dana was interested in this school because both her uncle and grandfather were alumni. Of all the schools Dana was evaluating, this one had the best academic reputation and the largest network of hospitals with multiple practice venues, and in preliminary conversations, it seemed likely to offer the largest scholarships. She also really liked the admission counselors she had talked to.

Dana had an appointment scheduled for next Friday with the admissions director for the nursing program. Dana had never taken a trip like this by herself. Most of her excursions in high school had been to the suburbs of this city or to smaller cities in the rural parts of the state. Even on these trips, she had always been with family or friends. Now her sister could not accompany her due to work, and her mother could not come because she had a dentist appointment for a routine check-up. Her mother refused to change the appointment, and Dana couldn't understand why. In truth, Dana was terrified of making this trip.

II

Ivan T. didn't know what to do. The summer after high school graduation had been difficult for him. His father had reappeared in his life and was claiming he had been sober for more than a year now. Because of his alcoholism, his father had been fired from several positions. With each firing, the caliber of job and pay had declined. Now, his father was working as a clerk at a big box store because it was the only job he could get. Ivan didn't believe his father was sober or trust him. He vowed he would never let his father disappoint or hurt him again.

Ironically, Ivan had started drinking to alleviate the stress. Several pictures of Ivan inebriated at a party had been posted on the Internet, and he knew he had made some incoherent and embarrassing tweets. Unfortunately, he had been caught and convicted of driving while intoxicated. It was a matter of public record. The attorney's fees and fines had cost more than $2,000, money he could ill afford to lose. The whole process had frightened him, and he would never forget the look on his mother's face. Although he will not admit it, Ivan liked the freedom and relaxation alcohol provided. However, for the last 6 months, Ivan had not touched alcohol.

Ivan knew that some of the professional schools he was applying to had specific questions on their applications that addressed criminal and reckless activities. He also knew that some schools were instituting criminal background checks. He wondered if the conviction would impact his licensure or job prospects.

III

Niki M. had narrowed her career choices to nursing, pharmacy, and physician assistant. Getting in a program, and one she wanted, would not be a problem. Scholarships and loans would not be difficult, either. Her undergraduate grades were very good, and her test scores on the respective admission exams ranked her in the top 10% of all students. Niki still had to make a choice as to which profession was likely to hold her interest. She knew that unless she was challenged, she would get bored. She knew that each profession offered pathways for postgraduate education.

Niki had always been at the top of her class both academically and athletically. But these rankings had been achieved with massive ancillary support from family and coaches. She had always been the "golden girl" for whom everything was easy. She had never had to take a part-time job, do her laundry, cook for someone, or deal with many of life's inconveniences. Now she was confronted with the task of funding her education, being massively in debt when she graduated, and having the energy to sustain herself through the program for at least 4 years and maybe more. How would she ever resolve the guilt over taking time away from her son? Although her parents were helpful, they were not indulgent or enabling. Their attitude was "you made this problem, now deal with it." Her father had put himself through night law school while holding a full-time job with a family to support. Niki knew that nothing in her previous experience could match this situation.

Niki considered how much easier it would be if she were still married. Even though her former husband had a relatively low-paying job, having his financial support would make things easier and he could help with the baby. Niki knew she still had some feelings for him.

IV

Ryan P. had just pulled on to the interstate. It was the early morning rush hour and cars were rushing by. He had to be on campus in 30 minutes because an exam was scheduled at the beginning of the hour. Ryan wanted at least 30 minutes to settle in and glance over his notes before the exam started. When he saw the dog, he knew he wouldn't make it on time.

There in the median was a German shepherd pup, clearly frightened and injured. The animal had obviously been hit by a car and had managed to make it to the side of the road. Ryan pulled over to help; he just couldn't leave the dog. It wasn't wearing a tag. Rather than driving his SUV, Ryan had his wife's car, a small mini-hybrid. Not only was the car small, but it was also full of shopping bags his wife had left in the car.

Ryan approached the dog with trepidation. He didn't know if the dog would try to bite him because of the pain. Luckily, the animal could sense that Ryan was there to help. He stroked the animal to calm it down and began to think how he was going to get it in the car and what he was going to do with it. The animal's hindquarters were bloody. He took his coat off and wrapped the animal in it. He could barely lift the animal by himself but managed to get it in the car after rearranging the packages. Ryan eased into the flow of traffic and began to consider what to do with the dog and what he would say to the instructor because he was going to miss the exam.

⫶ LEARNING OBJECTIVES

- Describe the model of professionalism.
- Discuss the elements of professionalism: accountability, altruism, duty, honor, integrity, excellence, and respect for others.

✦ KEY TERMS

- Accountability
- Altruism
- Deliberate practice
- Duty
- Excellence
- Honor and integrity
- Professionalism
- Respect for others

What Is a Profession?

ACCORDING TO CRUESS ET AL. (2004, p. 75), a profession is defined as follows:

> An occupation whose core element is work based on the mastery of a complex body of knowledge and skills. It is a vocation in which knowledge of some department of sciences or learning or the practice of an art founded upon it is used in the service of others. Its members are governed by codes of ethics and profess a commitment to competence, integrity and morality, altruism, and the promotion of the public good within their domain. These commitments form the basis of a social contract between a profession and society, which in return grants the profession a monopoly over the use of its knowledge base, the right to considerable autonomy in practice and the privilege of self-regulation. Professions and their members are accountable to those served and to society.

In short, a profession is characterized by:

- Mastery of a body of knowledge
- High levels of autonomy
- A code of behavior
- A social contract to do good for the individual and society

Who Is a Professional?

ANYONE WHO ADHERES TO THE standards of a profession and practices within that profession is a professional. "A real professional is a technician who cares" (Maister 1997, p. 16). Professionals are people who do the job on a day they do not want to, at a time they do not want to, with a patient or client they do not like, even though they might not get paid, because the patient or client needs help.

What Is Professionalism?

The first known usage of the term **professionalism** was in 1856. A working definition of professionalism that is precise and suitable across all professions and circumstances is elusive. Most of us have an intuitive sense of professionalism and are acquainted with someone who embodies this ideal. The lack of definitional clarity in discussing professionalism is reinforced by the number of frameworks and constructs similar to professionalism, including: professional ethics, professional commitment, professional responsibility, professional attitude, professional behavior, professional competence, professional values, professional identity/image, moral reasoning, work ethic, empathy, caring, advocacy, and covenantal relationships (Hammer et al. 2003).

Professionalism is a complex ensemble of values, attitudes, beliefs, and behaviors. The core values that define professionalism include: (1) a commitment to the highest standards of excellence in practice, (2) a commitment to the interest of patients; and (3) a commitment to the needs of the community.

The core values that define professionalism are elaborated as follows (Data from Board of Internal Medicine):

- **Accountability**—to individual patients in fulfilling the covenants of the patient–provider relationship; to society's health needs; and to the profession for honoring their codes of conduct.
- **Altruism**—the willingness to serve the best interest of the patient rather than your self-interest.
- **Excellence**—a conscientious commitment to improvement.
- **Duty**—a commitment to serve the patient even when it is inconvenient.
- **Honor and integrity**—a commitment to the highest standards of behavior.
- **Respect for others**—a belief in the value of all human beings, including patients, families, and other healthcare providers.

Professionalism also is an ethos (guiding beliefs and ideals that describe a community), an ethic, and an aspirational code for how to behave in a specific occupational role. Being professional constrains us in our choices and obligates us to behave in certain ways. Violation of those behaviors will be deemed as unprofessional. Think of professionalism as the religion of the specific professional group you are about to enter.

Accountability

"Accountability refers to the perception of defending or justifying one's conduct to an audience that has reward or sanction authority, and where rewards or sanctions are perceived to be contingent upon audience evaluation of such conduct" (Beu and Buckley 2001, p. 59). Accountability consists of the people accountable to one another, the areas of accountability, and the process by which people are held accountable.

People are held accountable by rules, codes of conduct, laws, and mechanisms of social control such as the expectations of important others. People also hold themselves individually accountable and suffer the pains of shame and guilt as a result. Healthcare professionals are responsible for the following (Data from Emanuel 1996):

- Reliable delivery of care.
- Quality of decision making.
- Confidentiality.
- Fiduciary obligations. Is the financial benefit of the patient paramount to ours?
- Responsibilities arising from patient vulnerability.
- Practitioner personal standards. Are we competent, and do we remain so?
- Equity. Are services delivered equitably?
- Cultural representation. Are we sensitive to diverse populations?
- Procedures for resolving disputes. Do they provide procedural and distributive justice?

Healthcare providers are responsible to individual patients, physicians, pharmacists, nurses, other healthcare providers, hospitals, managed care, professional associations, employers, private payers, government, investors, lawyers and courts, pharmaceutical companies, and other providers of health-related products.

Accountability can be viewed through three distinct lenses: (1) professional accountability, that of the provider and recipient of professional services; (2) economic accountability—as a consumer of healthcare as a product; and (3) political accountability—as a citizen concerned with a public good. Given the different focus of each perspective, conflict arises (Emanuel 1996). Tension also exists in the call for a "no blame" posture in the pursuit of error-free quality and the demand for accountability. The distinction between blameworthy and responsible is subtle but important (Wachter and Pronovost 2009). In other words, you may be responsible or accountable for an act, but if acting as a well-meaning professional who just made a mistake, you should not be considered blameworthy.

What Is Attribution Theory?

Attribution theory deals with how people justify their performance decisions. In other words, how do they explain the fact that they made a mistake? Accountability for positive outcomes is easy to assume. Accountability for negative outcomes is difficult. Accepting accountability for less than professional behavior, mistakes, errors, and deficiencies is difficult psychologically. True professionals willingly acknowledge and accept their part in subpar performance rather than blaming others—in short, they don't make excuses.

Accountability is a professional obligation. Accepting responsibility for deficient performance generates emotional reactions, cognitive assessments, and behavioral reactions. Following are some typical responses to accepting responsibility for deficient performance:

- Shame conjures feelings of inadequacy, self-contempt, embarrassment, self-exposure, and indignity.
- Guilt is a transitory, affective state arising from violating a standard. Guilt involves remorse, anxiety, and regret at having done something to hurt someone else.
- Self-reproach is punishment for a mistake. Self-reproach involves an excessive sense of personal responsibility. Those who reproach themselves hold to an impossible standard with little concern for capability, circumstances, or individual psychology.

From a psychological perspective, responsibility needs to be attributed accurately and realistically. "A clumsy focus on personal responsibility risks leading to self-defeating emotions like depression and overanxiety" (Nelson-Jones 1987, p. 7). It is critical that the offending party does not needlessly erode his or her self-worth. Accepting responsibility for a deficient performance is only valuable if it results in improved future performance. The best advice comes from a book on managing medical failure: when confronted with inadequate performance, *forgive and remember* (Bosk 1979).

Altruism

Altruism is characterized by seeking to increase the welfare of another person rather than yourself; it is voluntary, the intention is to help another, and no external reward is expected. In many instances, altruism contains an element of personal risk, for example, running into a burning building to save someone else's child. In the clinical arena, this is seldom the case.

Two mechanisms can explain altruistic behavior. The first is termed egoistic; engaging in altruistic behavior will make the person feel good and look good to others. In other words, the person gets something out of it. The second mechanism is pure altruism; the person wants to eliminate the suffering of other people without regard for his or her benefits.

Can altruism be learned? It can. The human brain is plastic. Brain growth and learning are possible over a lifetime. Training in compassion has been shown to increase altruistic behaviors (Weng et al. 2013). Also, as with any behavioral pattern, there is always a choice. His Holiness the Dalai Lama contends that people can either be compassionate or not; in the end, it is all personal choice. Quite simply, students can choose to be altruistic, just as they can choose not to cheat on a test.

Altruism does not require grand, life-risking behavior such as falling on a hand grenade. Simple, thoughtful gestures suffice, as when a nurse sits down to share a popsicle and intimate stories with a cancer patient to acknowledge and ease the nausea and discomfort of a chemotherapy treatment. As Mother Teresa observed, "I never will understand all the good that a simple smile can accomplish."

Most infants and small children are the center of their world and their parents' world. With maturity comes an understanding that you are no longer the center of the universe and that the selfish pursuit of personal happiness is futile. It is impossible to acquire enough attention and things to make yourself authentically happy. With maturity, the search for selfish fulfillment is replaced by an awareness of others' needs and your power to address these needs. Altruistic emotions and behaviors have been shown to positively impact mental health and physical health. "Altruism results in deeper and more positive social integration, distraction from personal problems and the anxiety of self-preoccupation, enhanced meaning and purpose as related to well-being, a more active lifestyle that counters cultural pressures toward isolated passivity, and the presence of positive emotions such as kindness that displace harmful negative emotions" (Post 2005, p. 70).

The Dark Side of Altruism

At the extreme, altruism may be pathological, leading to hyperempathy, compassion fatigue, codependency, animal hoarding, pathological certitude (believing you are acting in another's best interests, although you may not be), and enabling. Consider the physician who insists on heroic efforts to prolong the life of an individual who recognizes that the end is coming, who has made their peace, who has lived a good and full life, and who does not want to suffer any more. Such professionals believe they know what is best. They are compelled in their certitude of what they believe is the best interest of the patient and subject the individual to needless procedures, tests, and suffering. The belief regarding altruism that more is always better is simply not true. Professional decisions are always decisions about costs, benefits, and probabilities (Oakley et al. 2012). These decisions are tempered by judgment and wisdom, an understanding of what is important in life.

Also, individuals may engage in illegal or unethical behaviors if they believe others will benefit. For example, the Major League Baseball pitcher Andy Pettitte defended his use of human growth hormone, a banned substance, so as not to let his team down. Similarly, a researcher may shade his results in order to maintain funding for a department or to support his graduate students. A physician may perform questionable procedures if he or she believes the practice or hospital needs the funds to keep operating and preserve jobs (Gino, Ayal, and Ariely 2013).

Duty, Honor, and Integrity

Duties are obligations, in this case freely assumed. Honor is characterized by a keen sense of ethical conduct. Integrity is the quality of being honest and of expressing moral uprightness. Further, integrity implies wholeness.

For healthcare professionals, obligations of duty, honor, and integrity are integrated into the individual's behavior and expressed in all contexts. One cannot have integrity and be dutiful and honorable in one's dealing with patients while simultaneously defrauding insurance companies.

What Is a Virtue?

Morality is the set of rules, doctrines, and lessons that delineates right and wrong behavior. Morality offers a solution to solving the everyday problems of life. Virtue involves conforming to these standards. Virtues express themselves in exemplary conduct. Society values these characteristics. Some virtues are believed to be universal across all cultures, grounded in biology and selected in an evolutionary process that is important to the survival of the species. The six universal virtues are presumed to be wisdom, courage, humanity, justice, temperance, and transcendence (Peterson and Seligman 2004, p. 13).

Virtues and Character

Virtues are seated in character. Character is seen as the foundation of conduct. Individuals are born with some aspects of character, whereas other aspects develop over time. Character expresses the values and sensibilities of an individual. Good character results from an integration of personality traits organized around internalized moral values that are honed through practical application.

What Is Conscientiousness?

Conscientiousness is the psychological process or mechanisms for expressing the virtues of duty, honor, and integrity. Empirical work confirms this link (Murphy and Lee 1994; Moon 2001). Conscientiousness is the route to meeting the standard of duty, honor, and integrity. As a personality trait, conscientiousness is presumed to be relatively stable and general, but subject to variation due to circumstance. Consequently, the more practitioners exhibit conscientious behavior, the more likely they are to meet and exceed the professional threshold for duty, honor, and integrity. Conscientious professionals are seen as reliable, punctual, diligent, persistent, self-regulating, achievement oriented, methodical, trustworthy, accountable, self-disciplined, well organized, thorough, detail oriented, careful, and able to assess risk appropriately.

Self-Control as the Master Virtue

An aspect of conscientiousness involves self-control. To meet the professional obligation to duty, honor, and integrity, many impulses must be stifled. Lack of professionalism is often a deficiency in self-control. Some consider self-control the master virtue and the moral muscle (Baumeister and Exline 2000). The process of self-control involves three activities. The first is a clear understanding of the standards to be adhered to, the second is monitoring of the self (i.e., of keeping track of one's behavior), and the third is a capacity to alter behavior to conform to the standard.

Self-Control as a Limited Resource

Self-control has been likened to a moral muscle. The executive aspect of the self, the ability to make decisions, interrupt behaviors, and initiate behaviors, rests on strength of self-control. Keep in mind that self-control strength is limited; only so many impulses and urges can be constrained at one time. Undertaking a diet during study for a board exam is probably not a good choice. This explains why small annoyances under stress often result in inappropriate overreactions. A flat tire on the day of a final evokes a completely different response than a flat tire the day after graduation. Muscles fatigue with exercise; similarly, self-control fatigues with repeated use. Like a muscle, once rested, the ability to control oneself returns with rest. Also, like a muscle, repeated use of self-control increases self-control strength.

Excellence

For a professional, excellence is more than a state, it is a commitment to a career-long pursuit not only to be competent, but to exceed competence— to be more than the norm. In the pursuit of excellence, the individual may be motivated by two different goals. The first goal is a performance goal. A performance goal is about winning positive accolades and avoiding negative condemnations. In this context, achieved goals are measures of your ability. Conversely, not achieving these goals marks you as deficient. To defend their ego, individuals may shy away from tasks that seem beyond their level of competence. This approach is about appearing smart. The second goal is the focus on mastery of the task, of increasing competence. The second goal is a learning goal. With this approach, setbacks are seen as opportunities for learning rather than insurmountable obstacles. For a professional, excellence is the pursuit of superior patient care.

What Is Achievement Motivation?

Achievement motivation is a psychological process influencing individuals to strive to attain goals. Achievement motivation is a concept that encompasses several factors. Those factors are as follows (Data from Cassidy and Lynn 1989):

- **Work ethic:** originates from the concept of the Protestant work ethic and describes motivation to achieve based on the reinforcement the work itself provides. It is a desire to work hard.
- **Pursuit of excellence:** motivation that finds reward in performing to the best of one's ability.
- **Status aspiration:** motivation based on climbing the social ladder, to dominate, or to lead.
- **Competitiveness:** motivation based on enjoyment of the competition with a goal of winning.
- **Acquisition of money and wealth:** motivation based on material reward.
- **Mastery:** motivation based on competition with oneself.

Note that the pursuit of excellence, work ethic, and mastery are internal or intrinsic motivators, whereas status aspiration and the acquisition of money and wealth are obviously external.

How to Get Better?

There is no easy way to achieve excellence. Given a requisite base level of intellectual, moral, and personal intelligence, innate talent is probably not a deciding factor. What is important is a belief that improvement is possible. A deep belief in your ability to improve is the foundation. Next is a deep commitment to the process. Some have characterized this commitment as "rage to master" (Winner 1996, p. 271). It has to be something you really want, to the extent that you will sacrifice innumerable other things to get it. Commitment alone will not be sufficient; it has to be coupled with a specific type of practice termed **deliberate practice**. The most effective practice requires a well-defined task at an appropriate level of difficulty suited to the individual, informed feedback, and opportunities for repetition and correction. Deliberate practice is designed to improve performance. Deliberate practice requires high levels of mental concentration. Concentration is the critical element of deliberate practice. Deliberate practice may not necessarily be fun, although some individuals might find it or aspects of it enjoyable.

The Role of Willpower

Lifelong learning and the pursuit of excellence require discipline and the willingness to forgo immediate pleasures for long-term benefit that is often little rewarded or appreciated by others. Only you know if you have done the best you can in a situation. Only you know if you are working at less than your capacity. Although your performance appraisals may still be adequate or even glowing, only you know if it is your best work. Only you know if your skills are starting to erode.

Lifelong learning in the pursuit of excellence requires willpower. The potential to improve resides in our willpower. We can control our thoughts through willpower. We can use willpower to control our emotions, mood, and affect. Waking up grouchy does not mandate going to bed irritable. You are most likely to be as happy as you decide to be. We can use willpower to control our impulses, to resist the temptations that continuously offer enticing alternatives to the hard work of doing good and being good. Finally, willpower can be used to control our performance—specifically, focusing "energy on the task at hand, finding the right combination of speed and accuracy, managing time, [and] persevering when you feel like quitting" (Baumeister and Tierney 2011, p. 37). Empirical evidence confirms this about willpower: you have a finite amount of willpower that depletes as you use it, and the same reservoir of willpower is used for all tasks. Consequently, the caveat is that when you dip into the willpower reservoir, it is best to focus on only one task at a time. For most of us, it is not that we do not have goals, but that we have too many of them. Willpower is enhanced by a focus not on the minutia of the daily task, but on the prize at the end; not on laying the bricks, but on the cathedral that will result. Willpower is not about continuous denial; when markers are met on the path to excellence, self-rewards are in order. It is not masochism that is of interest, but continuous improvement.

Respect for Others

Respect is having a due regard for the feelings, rights, and wishes of another. The fact that someone is a person, no matter his or her status, conditions, or accomplishments, entitles that person to respect and the behaviors that emanate from that respect. With this respect, there is no comparison and no appraisal. This type of respect is due to all people and due to them equally. This is a universal obligation of all people toward one another. It is this type of respect that professionalism demands. Although this respect is universal, it does not mean that all people are treated the same because they vary in their needs and aspirations. In short, an unconditional valuing of patients as persons is the aspiration.

Respect for Patients Versus Respect for Others at Work

The standard for professionalism demands that all people encountered in the professional, clinical, and work context be respected. However, this demand varies by the individual and their position and circumstances. The expression of respect due a dying patient is different than that due the chief executive officer of the health system, the chief of medicine, a fellow practitioner, the administrative staff, technicians, and the driver delivering product into the building. Only with the patient does the practitioner have the unique covenantal obligation that professionalism demands. For the patient, the demand is to care; for the others, the demand is to be civil.

How Is Respect for Others Expressed in a Clinical Context?

Respect for others in a clinical context is expressed as (Data from Maloney 2009):

- Acceptance of patients as they are and where they are.
- Advocating for the rights of patients.
- Awareness of personal bias and the family and cultural dynamics at play.
- Caring—What can I do to help the patient through this?
- Collegiality—discussing with other practitioners what patients' feelings are and what they mean.
- Communicating clearly and appropriately with patients, both verbally and nonverbally.
- Compassion—a willingness to listen.

- Competence to ask the right questions and to assess the situation.
- Dignity—not taking patients' independence away and attention to privacy.
- Empathy—picturing patients' needs as primary and treating patients as you would want to be treated.
- Justice—health care is justice due the other; respect is about equality.
- Kindness—thinking about how you can help and having a sense of humor.
- Presence—being there with the patient and being humble.
- Reciprocity—viewing health care as a chance to give back all the good that has been given you.
- Reflection—taking time to think how you could have done it better.
- Relatedness—being able to engage with patients.
- Teaching—taking time to teach patients what they need to know.
- Time—not being rushed.
- Touch—a simple pat on the shoulder.

Advice on How to Treat People at Work

Some of the best advice on how to treat people is more than 75 years old. What follows borrows from that publication, *How to Win Friends and Influence People* by Dale Carnegie (1936). There is nothing wrong with wanting people at work to like you; things go smoother that way. The secrets to this are:

- Don't criticize, condemn, or complain.
- Give honest and sincere appreciation.
- Smile.
- Show respect.
- If wrong, admit it.
- See the other's point of view.

John Walter Wayland wrote in 1899 that a true man was one "who does not make the poor man conscious of his poverty, an obscure man of his obscurity, or any man of his inferiority or deformity: who is himself humbled if necessity compels him to humble another; who does not flatter wealth, cringe before power, or boast of his own possessions or achievements; who speaks with frankness but always with sincerity and sympathy; whose deed follows his word."

Conclusion

THIS CHAPTER PRESENTS A MODEL of professionalism characterized by the following attributes: accountability, altruism, duty, honor, integrity, excellence, and respect for others. It also discusses some of the underlying psychological processes associated with these attributes.

What Do the Practitioners/Others Say?

FOR NEXT CLASS, BE PREPARED to discuss professionalism or one of the attributes of professionalism based on any *one* of the following:

- A discussion with your colleagues, or others, on how they feel and what they know about being professional or the attribute of professionalism.
- An article on professionalism or the attribute of professionalism, either from the research literature or any other source.
- A movie, television program, or YouTube video about professionalism or the attribute of professionalism.
- A book on professionalism or the attribute of professionalism (literary, historical, psychological, or any other source).

Personal Learning Plan: Professionalism

USE THE FOLLOWING GUIDE TO develop a personal and professional growth project.

What prompted you to develop this plan?	
What is the general area for improvement?	
What is the specific issue for improvement?	
Why is this important to you?	
How do you generally act in these areas?	
What are your goals?	
What strategies are required?	
Who/what is necessary to meet your goals with this strategy?	
How will you measure success/failure with this effort?	
How will you reflect and capture the lesson from this effort that can be generalized to other circumstances?	

The Students: Personal and Professional Issues

BASED ON THE DESCRIPTION OF each student at the beginning of the chapter, what are the personal and professional issues (either immediately or in the future) confronting each student? Consider whether they are linked and, if so, how. Finally, what would you recommend to each student to resolve these issues?

Dana S.

Personal Issues

Professional Issues

Are They Linked? Will the Personal Issues Impact Professional Behavior?

Recommendations

Ivan T.

Personal Issues

Professional Issues

Are They Linked? Will the Personal Issues Impact Professional Behavior?

Recommendations

Niki M.

Personal Issues

Professional Issues

Are They Linked? Will the Personal Issues Impact Professional Behavior?

Recommendations

Ryan P.

Personal Issues

Professional Issues

Are They Linked? Will the Personal Issues Impact Professional Behavior?

Recommendations

Exercises

Accountability

1. Take a moment to consider whether the following statements describe you.

I believe I am in control of my circumstances.

I believe that others are in control of my circumstances.

It is easy for me to accept blame and admit mistakes.

I believe it is up to me to make myself happy.

I tend to feel sorry for myself.

I believe I am in control of my feelings.

I tend to meet all my obligations on time.

In group projects, I do my fair share.

I believe I am in control of my physical health.

I believe I am in control of my stress levels.

2. Based on your responses to these statements, write a one-paragraph description of yourself in relation to accountability.

3. With several of your classmates, discuss specific behaviors that indicate that a student or practicing professional is acting accountable for his or her actions.

Altruism

With several of your classmates discuss whether you believe potential students should be required to demonstrate altruistic attitudes, values, and behaviors for acceptance into your program. If so, how would you assess this? Write a one-paragraph summary of your discussion.

Duty, Honor, and Integrity

I am loath to close. We are not enemies, but friends. We must not be enemies. Though passion may have strained it must not break our bonds of affection. The mystic chords of memory, stretching from every battlefield and patriot grave to every living heart and hearthstone all over this broad land, will yet swell the chorus of the Union, when again touched, as surely they will be, by the better angels of our nature. (Abraham Lincoln, First Inaugural Address, March 4, 1861)

1. Faced with secession and the splitting of the Union, Lincoln closed his first inaugural address with the above quote. His appeal to prevent this dissolution rested on a belief in the "better angels of our nature," the best part of what it means to be human. He believed that ultimately this aspect of humanity would assert itself. Do you agree that there is a better part of human nature?

2. Do you believe it is better to die rich as a result of having stretched the obligations of duty, honor, and integrity (but not having done anything illegal) or to die less affluent but having adhered strictly to the obligations of duty, honor, and integrity?

Excellence

1. Given the appropriate attitude, commitment, and work, do you believe people can accomplish anything they want?

2. Review a time in your life and a circumstance where you pursued excellence. How did it turn out? What did you learn?

Respect for Others

Have you ever made fun of someone at work, said something hurtful, cursed at someone, been rude to someone, or gossiped about someone? If you answered yes to any of these, how did this make you feel? How did you handle it? How would you feel if someone did the same thing to you?

Professionalism

1. With several of your classmates, for each of the following components of professionalism, develop specific markers or behaviors that express that component. For example, respect for others could be expressed as showing up on time, dressing appropriately, and remembering names.

Accountability

1.

2.

3.

Altruism

1.

2.

3.

Duty, honor, and integrity

1.

2.

3.

Excellence

1.

2.

3.

Respect for others

1.

2.

3.

1. How do you rate yourself on these dimensions?

2. Write a one-page executive summary of the chapter.

3. Review the mind map from the opening of the chapter. Would you change anything after reading the chapter?

What's Important to You in the Chapter?

WITH SEVERAL OF YOUR CLASSMATES, discuss the idea or ideas that are most likely to effect a change in your values, attitudes, or behaviors. Be succinct. Write no more than two sentences. If Blackboard is used in your class, post your important ideas to the site.

References

Baumeister, R. F., and Exline, J. J. (2000). Self-control, morality, and human strength. *Journal of Social and Clinical Psychology.* 19 (1), 29–42.

Baumeister, R. F., and Tierney, J. (2011). *Wisdom.* New York, NY: Penguin Press.

Beu, D., and Buckly, M. R. (2001). The hypothesized relationship between accountability and ethical behavior. *Journal of Business Ethics.* 34, 57–73.

Board of Internal Medicine. (2001). *Project Professionalism, American Board of Internal Medicine,* Philadelphia, PA.

Bosk, C. L. (1979). *Forgive and Remember.* Chicago, IL: The University of Chicago Press.

Carnegie, D. (1936). *How to Win Friends and Influence People.* New York, NY: Simon & Schuster.

Cassidy, T., and Lynn, R. (1989). A multifactorial approach to achievement motivation: The development of a comprehensive measure. *Journal of Occupational Psychology.* 62, 301–312.

Cruess, S. R., Johnston, S., and Cruess, R. L. (2004). "Profession": A working definition for medical educators. *Teaching and Learning in Medicine.* 16 (1), 74–76.

Emanuel, L. L. (1996). A professional response to demands for accountability: Practical recommendations regarding ethical aspects of patient care. *Annals of Internal Medicine.* 124, 240–249.

Gino, F., Ayal, S., and Ariely, D. (2013). Self-serving altruism? The lure of unethical actions that benefit others. *Journal of Economic Behavior and Organization.* 93, 285–292.

Hammer, D. P., Berger, B. A., Beardsley, R. S., and Easton, M. R. (2003). Student professionalism. *American Journal of Pharmaceutical Education.* 67 (1/4), 544–572.

Maister, D. H. (1997). *True Professionalism.* New York, NY: Touchstone.

Maloney, R. J. (2009). A phenomenological focus on Levinas' concept of alterity interpreted as respect for the other in a healthcare encounter. Unpublished dissertation. Widener University.

Moon, H. (2001). Two faces of conscientiousness: Duty and achievement striving in escalation of commitment dilemmas. *Journal of Applied Psychology.* 86 (3), 533–540.

Murphy, K. R., and Lee, S. L. (1994). Personality variables related to integrity test scores: The role of conscientiousness. *Journal of Business and Psychology*. 8 (4), 413–424.

Nelson-Jones, R. (1987). *Personal Responsibility Counseling and Therapy: An Integrative Approach*. Cambridge, MA: Hemisphere Publishing.

Oakley, B., Knafo, A., Madhavan, G., and Wilson, D. S., eds. (2012). *Pathological Altruism*. Oxford, United Kingdom: Oxford University Press.

Peterson, C., and Seligman, M. E. P. (2004). *Character Strengths and Virtues*. Oxford, United Kingdom: Oxford University Press.

Post, S. G. (2005). Altruism, happiness and health: It's good to be good. *International Journal of Behavioral Medicine*. 12 (2), 66–77.

Wachter, R. M., and Pronovost, P. J. (2009). Balancing "no blame" with accountability in patient safety. *New England Journal of Medicine*. 361, 1401–1406.

Weng, H. Y., Fox, A. S., Shackman, A. J., Stodola, D. E., Caldwell, J. Z. K., Olson, M. C., Rogers, G. M., and Davidson, R. J. (2013) Compassion training alters altruism and neural response to suffering. *Psychological Science*. http://pss.sagepub.com/content/early/2013/05/20/095679761 2469537.

Winner, E. (1996). The rage to master: The decisive role of talent in the visual arts. In *Road to Excellence*. K. Anders Ericsson, ed. Mahwah, NJ: Lawrence Erlbaum Associates.

CHAPTER
3

Psychology of
Professionalism

Preassessment: Psychology of Professionalism

Mind Mapping

*Consider the phrase displayed on the page. For this phrase, without thinking or editing, write down the ideas, concepts, examples, contradictions, and theories that come to mind. Do not arrange them in any systematic or orderly manner. Scatter them about the page. Now, draw lines between your additions, indicating that there is a relationship between the terms. If something causes something else, indicate this with an arrow. Relationships may be reciprocal, meaning both cause each other, requiring arrows at both ends. Indicate the strength of the relationships by darkening and thickening the lines; stronger relationships have darker and thicker lines. **Most important: There is no right answer. Do not compare with your classmates.** What you have is a mind map, your mental representation of these topics. Review to determine if anything has changed following this section.*

Reasons for Being Professional

The Students

I

DANA S.'S MOTHER GREW UP in an earlier generation. Her mother had been raised to consider refinement, manners, and gentility of spirit as virtues. Dana was always shocked while staying with friends' families; some of her friends' mothers were raucous, direct, and explicit, and some couples were confrontational and seemed to relish it.

Dana blushed easily and profusely. She didn't like conflict or discussion about ideas where people didn't agree. She really didn't like being singled out for her opinion. At parties and social gatherings, she was content to stay on the sidelines, and if with a date, she would stay in his shadow to avoid the limelight. Being called on in class or asked to present was excruciating.

Some of Dana's most vivid memories and emotional anchors were of her parents' arguments behind closed bedroom doors. She was surprised and troubled over how vitriolic and mean-spirited they were. Sometimes the arguments were so loud they would wake her up. This seemed to always happen when her father had just returned from a business trip. It was clear that in these circumstances her mother was not passive or refined. She had heard her mother curse her father on numerous occasions. Sometimes she would sneak down the hall and listen outside the door. She could hear every word. The names of other women kept coming up, women Dana did not know. One night, she heard her father threaten to leave. Although her mother had a degree, she had never worked, having always been a stay-at-home mom. Now when the arguments started, Dana just pulled the blankets up over her head.

II

Ivan T. found it ironic that, given the problems both he and his father had with alcohol, he was now tending bar. Ivan found that he had a natural affinity for small talk and could, when required, feign interest in the most banal of customers and stories. This skill resulted in Ivan making serious money in tips while working. This skill with the customers kept them drinking; Ivan was greatly appreciated by his manager. Ivan always got the best shifts and could get all the hours he wanted. Many weeks, Ivan found himself working over 40 hours. Ivan liked the money. It was the first time in his life when he had more than enough money in his pocket. The money allowed him to support a fairly lavish student lifestyle.

Ivan couldn't wait to graduate. He couldn't wait to make a full salary. He knew he would work all the hours he could. He also knew that when he graduated, there were always little "side deals" going on where extra money could be made. In his early clinical rotations, Ivan had been fortunate enough to meet a practitioner who seemed to have a very affluent lifestyle. Although the practitioner had not been explicit, he had alluded to some of these "side deals" as the source of his real income. The practitioner always complemented Ivan on his way with the patients and how they all liked him. Ivan knew that he would never be poor once he graduated; he had never forgotten the stigma of the reduced financial circumstances when his father had left.

Ivan had a more immediate problem. His grades had been gradually eroding over the past year as his hours at work had increased. In one course, he had to score an 85 on the final to pass. If he didn't, he would have to retake the course, possibly delaying his graduation.

III

Niki M. did not suffer fools gladly, even more so now that her time was so constrained with a child and school. Group assignments drove her crazy. She felt like she always carried the weaker students. Often, she simply did the work herself and presented it as already being done. Interestingly, some students resented this. Niki thought they would all appreciate it. During group discussions, she dominated the conversations and controlled the flow of the meetings. Students who disagreed with her were curtly shut off with the comment, "We don't have time for this." In Niki's mind, performance was the only objective; feelings didn't matter.

Lately, Niki found herself in the bathroom at school crying. On the way home from school last week, she had to pull over as she began to sob. Niki resented her mother for getting to be a stay-at-home mom. Why had her life turned out like this?

The one bright spot was her new relationship. He was charming and handsome and good with her son. He made her feel good and made her life easy. What was strange was that he was only available during the week and never on weekends. Niki sensed there was something mysterious about his life.

IV

Generally, Ryan P. was easy going about most things. He understood that sometimes in life situations needed to be endured in the pursuit of larger goals. Today's classes had tested his endurance. A new biochemistry professor had just been hired. It was clear that the professor's future was going to be in research, not in the classroom. In Ryan's second class that day, the instructor had "gone off" on a student who would not put his cell phone away. Although the material was boring, the aftermath of the instructor calling the student an idiot in front of all the other students was not. The students were incensed. Ryan was not. He felt the student deserved it. Ryan would have called him worse. He couldn't wait until tomorrow to hear what was going to happen.

After a hard day at school, Ryan came home to find his youngest daughter on the couch sobbing uncontrollably. Whatever had happen, it was clear his daughter felt badly about it. And there was his wife, screaming at her. She was holding a note from the school. His daughter had been caught plagiarizing a paper from the Internet for one of her classes. Ryan caught the last of the screaming match, "How could you do this to us? You have embarrassed us in front of all our friends and neighbors after all we have sacrificed for you!" It was not clear how long this had been going on, but it seemed like it had been for some time. Ryan started to get everyone to calm down. Ryan's wife turned to him and said, "You handle this; I can't talk to her. All I get from her is attitude." Up until that moment, Ryan had been most concerned about how he was going to pay their taxes. Now, he had to deal with this.

ⵚ LEARNING OBJECTIVES

Describe the psychology associated with professionalism. Specifically, the following:

- The motivation to act professionally
- Professional sensitivity
- Professional judgment
- Implementation of professional choices

❖ KEY TERMS

- Implementing professional choices
- Professional judgment
- Professional motivation
- Professional sensitivity
- Schema
- Tacit knowledge

CHAPTER 2 DECLARED THAT THE core values of professionalism (commitment to the highest standards of excellence in practice and commitment to the interest of the patients and community) are accountability, altruism, duty, excellence, honor, integrity, and respect for others. This chapter presents the psychology of professionalism, defined as (1) the sensitivity to professional situations, (2) the motivation to act professionally, (3) professional judgment, and (4) the ability to implement professional choices. Essentially, a content and process model for professionalism has been presented. To understand the psychology of professionalism is to understand the thoughts and feelings of the individual related to the topic and to consider factors in the environment that impact those thoughts and feelings. As with the content aspect of professionalism, it makes no sense to ask an inexperienced 20-year-old to discern an appropriate professional response to a situation, and then act accordingly, without first arming that person with a basic understanding of his or her underlying psychology. It is an unfair expectation to believe that the person will arrive at this information intuitively or informally, and it is a waste of time and resources to ask the person to do this when the elements of this process are known and readily available.

What Is the Psychology of Professionalism?

THE MODEL USED IN THIS work to explain the psychology of professionalism is derived from work by James Rest and Darcia Narvaez (Narvaez and Rest 1995; Rest and Narvaez 1994) and is composed of the following elements and assumptions. The model they present focuses on the psychology of moral development. The elements of that model translate to professionalism.

In describing the model here, the word *professional* is used as a direct substitute for the word *moral* that appears in the original work and is modified to be applicable to this context. The four dimensions of the model are:

Professional motivation—What priority does the individual assign to professional obligations relative to other choices? What causes someone to act professionally?

Professional sensitivity—the perception and interpretation of situations requiring a professional response, what is possible, what is required, who will be affected, and how they will react.

Professional judgment—identifying potential courses of action and selecting the most appropriate.

Implementing professional choices—what skills, courage, and tacit knowledge are required to carry out the appropriate professional choice.

These four psychological aspects depict an ensemble of processes. No single aspect is predictive of professional behavior. Each of the four aspects involves different kinds of cognitive–affective interactions with no cognitions without emotions, no emotions without cognition, and no professional behavior distinct from the underlying cognitions and affect. It is not suggested that these psychological aspects occur in the order detailed above. Rather, they interact with one another.

The psychology of professionalism is complex, multilayered, multifactorial, subtle, and nuanced. A convenient lens for understanding the psychology of professionalism (the four process elements detailed above) and professionalism in general is the **schema**—the mental blueprint of what professionalism is and how it is applied. Unlike many aspects of individual psychology, mental blueprints, or schemas, are accessible and amenable to being changed. In fact, the objective of this chapter and Chapter 2 is to provide the student with a more sophisticated mental blueprint of what it means to be professional.

Schemas

SCHEMAS ARE COGNITIVE STRUCTURES REPRESENTING individuals' beliefs and assumptions about themselves and the world. They are mental representations of what is going on, blueprints, scripts, models, narratives, or theories of the world. "Schemas are powerful tools.... They guide perception, attention, decisions, habits, and behavior" (Narvaez and Bock 2002, p. 304).

All students come with naïve schemas about professionalism gleaned from their past experience. They also come with schemas about integrity, duty, honor, themselves, others, altruism, and accountability. It is the task of the school to enrich those schemas. These naïve schemas serve as the scaffolding to which the mandates of professionalism, derived through experience at school and in practice, are arrayed. In other words, each student knows something about professionalism when they enter school. With experience, they should learn something more. The distribution of a professional code of conduct on matriculation is a first attempt to alter that schema. No matter what the school does, certain schemas are not likely to be changed in school. If one has an unshakable belief that patients are primarily commercial opportunities, no amount of proselytizing for professional conduct is likely to be effective. More specifically:

- Schemas lend structure to experience. Schema are activated from long-term memory in response to a new circumstance. The order and relationships among the elements of the existing schema are imposed on the new circumstance.
- Schemas determine the information that will be encoded and retrieved from memory.
- Schemas affect processing time, speed of information flow, and speed of problem solving. Schemas affect the speed of inferences about dilemmas.
- Schemas permit the observer to fill in missing data when data are missing or ambiguous.
- Schemas provide a basis for problem solving. Schemas provide a basis for interpreting the world. This interpretation drives the course of action and decision making.
- Schemas provide a basis for evaluating experience. People with highly developed schemas make more confident evaluations of situations.
- Schemas provide a basis for making plans, establishing goals, and developing behavioral routines to accomplish objectives (Data from Narvaez and Mitchell 2000).

In short, the idea of a schema is used as the lens for the psychology of professionalism. Schemas are the conduits for individuals to understand their particular psychology regarding professionalism. Discussion of the four psychological aspects of professionalisms follows. The influence of schemas on each aspect is considered in the exercises at the end of the chapter. The mind mapping exercise that begins each chapter is an exercise in surfacing schemas about that topic.

Professional Motivation

PROFESSIONAL MOTIVATION IS THE LINK between the ability to perceive that a situation requires a professional response and acting on that response. For any professional, there are always multiple external pressures and internal conscious and unconscious factors modified by the situation that impact the decision to act. Those pressures may include career, money, family, expediency, prejudice, ignorance, inexperience, emotional state, cognitive frame, indifference, hedonism, and so on. The question then is: Why does an individual choose to act professionally? What motivates an individual to act in accord with the highest demands of the profession?

- Practitioners are motivated to act professionally out of a fear of punishment and negative feedback because they are coerced or told to by someone in power.
- Practitioners are motivated to act professionally to avoid feeling shame, fear, or guilt.
- Practitioners are motivated to act professionally to maintain good relationships with individuals and with the larger community as a whole as a way of maintaining a practice.
- Practitioners are motivated to act professionally because it feels good.
- Practitioners are motivated to act professionally because it confirms their self-identity.
- Practitioners are motivated to act professionally out of a sense of ethical obligation, an understanding of the basic rights of individuals, and a concern for universal justice and fairness.

Professional Sensitivity

PROFESSIONAL SENSITIVITY IS A COMPLEX phenomenon of perception and interpretation. Perception includes attraction, empathy, attention, and mood. Perception of professional issues is semi-conscious or unconscious. Attentiveness is a key requirement for perception (Jagger 2011). Interpretation is the ability to determine that there is an issue that requires evaluation, to identify the professional issues embedded in a particular circumstance, and to interpret what actions are possible, who will be affected by those actions, and how those involved might be affected. Professional interpretation requires cultivation and learning. The sophistication and comprehensiveness of currently held professional schemas are critical to discerning the professional issues inherent in any situation.

Recognizing professional issues from the mass of environmental cues impinging on a professional requires selective attention, encoding, and recall of professional related stimuli. Cues that are most likely to be encoded are those that resonate with existing schemas for the situation. Schemas provide the scaffolding for assimilating new information. Schemas aid in recall and in structuring memory and help to edit unimportant and irrelevant information. Existing schemas are critical elements of professional sensitivity.

Social perception, or social cognition, is the ability to attend to and interpret social cues, language, paralinguistic information (intonation), and nonverbal signals (e.g., facial expressions, body language, gestures). Social perception also includes the ability to identify the emotions of others based on facial and vocal cues; the ability to attribute mental states of others, such as thoughts, beliefs, desires, and intentions; and conversational inference, which is the meaning that is derived from language based on context (McDonald 2011). Professional sensitivity also involves the ability to see the larger context of a situation.

Perception of social issues is affected by characteristics associated with the event. Those characteristics include frequency, intensity, size, novelty, the medium or cognitive process through which the event is received, and the perceiver. In particular, intensity influences decision making (May and Pauli 2002). Intensity is a function of the magnitude of the consequences of a situation, the consensus that a proposed act is good or evil, the probability that an act will actually happen and will actually result in the anticipated consequences, the length of time between the decision and the onset of consequences, the proximity of the decision maker for beneficiaries of the choice, and the number of people affected by the act. Think of the end-of-life choices facing a decision maker for a 95-year-old patient with cancer versus the end-of-life choices for a decision maker for a sitting American president who was the victim of an assassination attempt.

Professional Judgment

P ROFESSIONAL JUDGMENT CAN BE CONSIDERED from two perspectives. The first is straight forward and is synonymous with decision making. In other words, how does the practitioner make the choice to act professionally? Human decisions can be guided by logic (the pursuit of truth, maintaining consistency across beliefs, and solve syllogisms), probability (performing inductive inferences, dealing with samples of information involving error rather than full information that is error free, and making risky bets), and heuristics (rules of thumb that are fast and frugal, that satisfice rather than optimize, and that use limited amounts of information). No single approach is suitable in all circumstances. Heuristics are best employed in situations where a problem is computationally impossible, the future is uncertain, and the goals are ambiguous (Gigerenzer 2008), which is an apt description for many of the professional dilemmas a practitioner is confronted with. Thus, many professional choices are best understood as an application of fast and frugal heuristics (Gigerenzer 2008). Heuristics allow a practitioner to make decisions on the spot in real time (fast) and devoid of an extensive information search often not permitted by time (frugal). The heuristics underlying professional choice are generally unconscious. In one view, people have intuitions about moral choices anchored in emotions and then apply reasoning after the fact to justify a choice (Haidt 2001). An example of a professional heuristic is to treat everyone as if they were members of your own family.

The second perspective on professional judgment is more nuanced. Most professions subscribe to an ideal of technical rationality that relies on objectivity and detachment in pursuit of extracting generalizable findings and developing standard procedures. The uniqueness of circumstances is shunted aside in pursuit of the common denominators. This approach is, at heart, rational, scientific, evidence-based practice. Technical rationality is at the heart of the scientific method and the understanding and control of the physical, chemical, and many aspects of the biological world. Technical rationality anchors clinical judgment.

Practitioners, however, operate in what has been termed by Donald Schon as the "swampy lowlands" of practice. In other words, practice is messy, situations are novel, and the outcomes are ill-defined or, if defined, the outcomes may be in conflict. It is the computer programmer's dilemma of do you want the project on time, or right, or on budget—pick any two. It is in the "swampy lowlands" of practice where the human variable (not as the object of the choice, but as integral to the choice and its implementation) is considered. Clinical judgment is about improving the life of a human being. Professional judgment is about whether that quest is appropriate, whether the humans involved are aids or impediments, and how that quest is best structured and conducted.

Much of practice is routine. The accepted protocols suffice. However, some aspects of practice are the equivalent of a fifteenth-century mariner sailing off the known map to an uncharted place characterized only as "there be dragons." Where protocols fail to enlighten is where judgment intervenes. Judgment is the "ability to actuate knowledge with relevance, appropriateness, or sensitivity to context" (Dunne 1999, p. 710). Without judgment, professional practice is merely technical work. This is a more nuanced view of judgment than that of the straightforward decision making detailed earlier.

Implementation

RECOGNIZING A PROFESSIONAL DILEMMA, VALUING professionalism as a personal core value, and being able to determine a preferred professional choice are nothing without the ability, skills, and tacit knowledge to implement those choices. It is one thing to know that a department head or senior clinician is making a mistake but quite something else to take that person on and to know how to do it. Numerous skills and personal characteristics could be used in implementing any single professional choice.

There are two kinds of knowledge. There is the knowledge that can be verbalized, such as facts and concepts. There is also knowledge that cannot be verbalized, such as intuition and the knowledge of procedures. It is the difference between knowing what and knowing how. Our interest is in knowing how; specifically, how to implement a professional decision or judgment. In the clinical healthcare environment, there is the science of practice and the art of practice. The type of information that cannot be verbalized and is often the knowledge of "how to" is termed **tacit knowledge**. Healthcare practices tend to have clearly defined protocols for many circumstances that

are explicit and known by everyone. However, when to apply those protocols may be fuzzy and vary by institution or circumstance. It is the when to
apply that represents the tacit knowledge. Tacit knowledge about how to get
things done can only be learned through experience. The acquisition of tacit
knowledge requires that the practitioner reflect on circumstances and draw
the appropriate conclusions about how to behave. An important aspect of
tacit knowledge is understanding how all those affected by the choice will
react. Although it may be a correct choice, if an individual can sabotage that
choice, then another course of action is warranted.

Similar to the idea of tacit knowledge and useful in implementing professional decisions is the idea of practical intelligence—the ability to cope with
the challenges and opportunities of life (Albrecht 2007, p. 41). Some would
consider tacit knowledge and practical intelligence synonymous. Related
to these terms is the idea of behavioral social intelligence, the ability to be
effective in social situations.

Taken together, tacit knowledge, practical intelligence, and behavioral
social intelligence capture something that is critical in implementing professional choices—common sense. Common sense is the ability to solve problems in the real world. If your car breaks down in the desert, a mechanic
is probably a better companion to have than an automotive engineer. The
former can get the car running, whereas the latter might be able to tell you
why the car runs. People high in these attributes have the "street smarts" to
be effective and know how to lubricate the procedural, organizational, and
human gears to get things done.

Some professional choices may be controversial and run counter to
entrenched stakeholders. What may be required is the courage to implement those choices. "Courage entails the exercise of will to accomplish goals
in the face of opposition, either external or internal" (Peterson and Seligman
2004, p. 199). Courage is multifaceted. It can be a virtue, a state of mind, an
attitude, an emotion, a force, or an action (Yang, Milliren, and Blagen 2010).
Courage is not the absence of fear, but the ability to function despite fear.
Courage can also be thought of as bravery, perseverance in pursuit of goals,
authenticity and honesty, and vigor and enthusiasm. Courage is the use of
willpower to support one's beliefs; it is the psychological muscle that powers
moral choice. Courage is the mental strength that allows one to persevere in
the presence of adversity. It takes courage to confront a grieving family following a mistake that killed a family member; it takes courage to confront a

powerful clinician who may be slipping into senility; and it takes courage to risk your job to expose a financial scandal within an organization. Courage may require an overt act or require doing nothing in the face of pressure. Individual courage is relatively stable but malleable. Aristotle believed courage was a habit that formed through repetition. Professionalism without the courage to act is an academic exercise; it is wishful thinking.

Conclusion

THIS CHAPTER PRESENTED THE PSYCHOLOGY of professionalism as a process model. The psychology of professionalism requires a sensitivity to the professional aspects of a situation, the motivation to act professionally, the utilization of professional judgment, and the ability to implement professional choices.

What Do the Practitioners/Others Say?

FOR NEXT CLASS, BE PREPARED to discuss professional judgment based on any *one* of the following:

- A discussion with your colleagues, or others, on how they feel and what they know about professional judgment.
- An article on professional judgment, either from the research literature or any other source.
- A movie, television program, or YouTube video about professional judgment.
- A book on professional judgment (literary, historical, psychological, or any other source).

Personal Learning Plan: Psychology of Professionalism

USE THE FOLLOWING GUIDE TO develop a personal learning plan for yourself to improve an aspect of your professionalism.

What prompted you to develop this plan?	
What is the general area for improvement?	
What is the specific issue for improvement?	
Why is this important to you?	
How do you generally act in these areas?	
What are your goals?	
What strategies are required?	
Who/what is necessary to meet your goals with this strategy?	
How will you measure success/failure with this effort?	
How will you reflect and capture the lesson from this effort that can be generalized to other circumstances?	

The Students: Personal and Professional Issues

BASED ON THE DESCRIPTION OF each student at the beginning of the chapter, what are the personal and professional issues (either immediately or in the future) confronting each student? Consider whether they are linked and, if so, how. Finally, what would you recommend to each student to resolve these issues?

Dana S.

Personal Issues

Professional Issues

Are They Linked? Will the Personal Issues Impact Professional Behavior?

Recommendations

Ivan T.

Personal Issues

Professional Issues

Are They Linked? Will the Personal Issues Impact Professional Behavior?

Recommendations

Niki M.

Personal Issues

Professional Issues

Are They Linked? Will the Personal Issues Impact Professional Behavior?

Recommendations

Ryan P.

Personal Issues

Professional Issues

Are They Linked? Will the Personal Issues Impact Professional Behavior?

Recommendations

Exercises

Mindfulness

1. Mindfulness is a psychological process where the individual is aware of his or her thoughts, emotions, physical sensations, and environment in the moment. The process is nonjudgmental and accepting of what is. Mindfulness is a conscious choice. It is deliberate. To understand whether you are sensitive to professional situations, motivated to act professionally, make good professional judgments, and have the ability to implement professionalism requires that you be mindful. Mindfulness can be practiced and developed. As an exercise, set a timer for 3 minutes, and then record all your thoughts. Write just a word or two that represents the thought. Repeat the process with your emotions. Use the questions below as an aid to mindfulness about the psychological aspects of being a professional (McKay, Wood, and Brantley 2007; Keng, Smoski, and Robins 2011).

2. Privately consider what you believe the role of your instructors is in (1) the educational process and (2) your development as a professional. Having done this, discuss your answers with several of your classmates. If you adopted a different belief about what you believe your instructors' role to be, would it change your behavior in class, toward preparation, or toward them personally?

3. Do you believe it is more important to (1) get the highest grade possible or (2) master the material? If this belief changed, how would this impact your behavior?

4. Would you be willing to go against your clinical supervisor if you believed it would benefit the patient? What if you believed this might compromise your annual performance review?

5. When you think about the people you will treat in practice, notice the word you use to describe them. Is it patient, client, customer, or something else? How might this characterization affect how you treat them?

6. Do you believe that people on Medicaid should be viewed as the "deserving poor" or as "takers"? Do you treat patients on Medicaid differently than those covered by private insurance?

7. Is there a class of patients you routinely have a problem with? Why is this so?

8. If you find a patient physically attractive, have you ever looked at their files for their personal information and to find out where they live?

9. Write a one-page executive summary of the chapter.

10. Review the mind map from the opening of the chapter. Would you change anything after reading the chapter?

What's Important to You in the Chapter?

WITH SEVERAL OF YOUR CLASSMATES, discuss the idea or ideas that are most likely to effect change in your values, attitudes, or behaviors. Be succinct. Write no more than two sentences.

References

Albrecht, K. (2007). *Practical Intelligence.* San Francisco, CA: John Wiley & Sons.

Dunne, J. (1999). Professional judgment and the predicaments of practice. *European Journal of Marketing.* 33 (7/8), 707–719.

Gigerenzer, G. (2008). Moral intuition = fast and frugal heuristics? In *Moral Psychology, Vol. 2.* W. Sinnott-Armstrong, ed. Cambridge, MA: MIT Press.

Haidt, J. (2001). The emotional dog and its rational tail: A social intuitionist approach to moral judgment. *Psychological Review.* 108 (4), 814–834.

Jagger, S. (2011). Ethical sensitivity: A foundation for moral judgment. *Journal of Business Ethics Education.* 8, 13–30.

Keng, S., Smoski, M. J., and Robins, C. J. (2011). Effects of mindfulness on psychological health: A review of empirical studies. *Clinical Psychology Review.* 31 1041–1056.

May, D. R., and Pauli, K. P. (2002). The role of moral intensity in ethical decision making. *Business and Society.* 41 (1), 84–117.

McDonald, S. (2011). New frontiers in neuropsychological assessment: Assessing social perception using a standardized instrument: The Awareness of Social Inference Test. *Australian Psychologist.* 47, 39–48.

McKay, M., Wood, J. C., and Brantley, J. (2007). *The Dialectical Behavior Therapy Skills Workbook.* Oakland, CA: New Harbinger Publications.

Narvaez, D., and Bock, T. (2002). Moral schemas and tacit judgment or how the defining issues tests is supported by cognitive science. *Journal of Moral Education*, 31 (3), 297–314.

Narvaez, D., and Mitchell, C. (2000). Schemas, culture, and moral texts. In *Moral Education and Pluralism.* London, United Kingdom: Falmer Press.

Narvaez, D., and Rest, J. (1995). Four components of acting morally. In *Moral Development: An Introduction* (pp. 385–400). Boston, MA: Allyn and Bacon.

Peterson, C., and Seligman, M. E. P. (2004). *Character Strengths and Virtues.* Oxford, United Kingdom: Oxford University Press.

Rest, J. R., and Narvaez, D. (1994). Background: Theory and research. In *Moral Development in the Professions* (pp. 1–26). Hillsdale, NJ: Lawrence Erlbaum Associates.

Yang, J., Milliren, A., and Blagen, M. (2010). *The Psychology of Courage.* New York, NY: Routledge.

Suggested Readings

Gigerenzer, G. (2008). Why heuristics work. *Perspectives on Psychological Science.* 3 (1), 20–29.

Sternberg, R. J., and Horvath, J. A. (1999). *Tacit Knowledge in Professional Practice.* New York, NY: Routledge.

CHAPTER
4

The Dark Side

Preassessment: Impressions

Mind Mapping

Consider the term displayed on the page. For this term, without thinking or editing, write down the ideas, concepts, examples, contradictions, and theories that come to mind. Do not arrange them in any systematic or orderly manner. Scatter them about the page. Now, draw lines between your additions, indicating that there is a relationship between the terms. If something causes something else, indicate this with an arrow. Relationships may be reciprocal, meaning both cause each other, requiring arrows at both ends. Indicate the strength of the relationships by darkening and thickening the lines; stronger relationships have darker and thicker lines. **Most important: There is no right answer. Do not compare with your classmates.** *What you have is a mind map, your mental representation of these topics. Review to determine if anything has changed following this section.*

Evil

The Students

I

DANA S. WAS REALLY ENJOYING her rotations. She liked being out on the floor, interacting with patients, professional staff, and other residents and students doing their clinical work. Dana really just liked people. She even enjoyed talking to housekeeping and other support staff when she was on the elevator. She liked hearing about their children and their experiences, which were so much different from hers.

Dana always looked forward to lunch in the cafeteria. A group of residents, interns, and students from various specialties started to congregate at a big table in the corner. There was always someone there to talk to and discuss things. The conversation included the usual complaints and laments about their lives along with speculation about what life would be like after graduation. Dana particularly looked forward to lunch when one of the new pharmacy residents was in attendance. She found him attractive and kind. She mentioned one day that she had been having headaches and was sore from having fallen on the ice. He asked Dana to leave with him and stop by the pharmacy and he would get her some ibuprofen samples. When he checked the samples, there wasn't any ibuprofen, so he went to the shelf and gave her four tablets from the bottle on the shelf. This happened 3 days in a row, partly because she was still sore and having headaches but also partly because she wanted an excuse to stop by the pharmacy.

For years, since she was about 12 years old, Dana would have difficulty falling asleep as she reviewed her transgressions for the day. Dana was extremely conscientious and rule oriented. When she was a little girl, her mother wouldn't let her have candy before noon. To this day, Dana had a hard time eating a piece of candy in the morning. Recently, Dana was having a harder time falling asleep as she obsessed over the fact that she might be viewed as stealing medications from the pharmacy.

II

Ivan T. remembered when the father of one of his classmates had died. He remembers how much his friend talked about missing his father. Ivan felt nothing after his father died. The closest thing Ivan had to feelings about his death was relief. The focus of much of his anger and resentment was gone. Ivan had a suspicion that he had used the circumstance of his father abandoning the family as a justification for some of his past choices. Because life had been hard growing up for him, Ivan believed he was owed certain things. When he compared his circumstances with his friends, he knew he deserved some special consideration. Ivan thought this might be the reason for how he had handled some of his grade issues.

Ivan had been made executor for his father's estate, which was probably only about $5,000. Most of the little money his father had when he moved in had gone for medical expenses not covered by insurance. Ivan's father had received Social Security disability payments from the government for the last year of his life. Ivan needed to notify Social Security of his father's death so that the payments would cease. While filling out the paper work, Ivan turned on the local news. Apparently a believed long-lived local resident had really not lived that long after all; the family had neglected to file the death notice and collected payments for the past 27 years. The amount was sizeable.

If Ivan was honest with himself, he always felt his father owed him something. If he couldn't get it while he was alive, Ivan thought it only fair that in death he would get it from his father. Ivan decided he would wait 6 months to file the death notice and use the continued payments to pay his tuition for next semester. Given the money the federal government wasted and the amount withheld each paycheck for Social Security, Ivan had no qualms about this.

III

Things were great for Niki M. If she felt alone at school, she would get her phone out and watch videos. Being in the program always made her feel good about herself and what having the degree would mean for the both her and her son. Niki wasn't sure, but she thought she was picking up "vibes" whenever she had to meet with her 40-year-old professor. Six more weeks and she would be out of his class, with no other classes with him for the rest of the program. He was very attractive but only just her height, and she had always only liked tall men. Also, she had picked up a part-time job reading and editing faculty grants and papers before final submission. It was easy and convenient work. She could do it late at night when the baby was asleep, and it let her use some of the skills and talents from her undergraduate English degree.

When editing the grants and papers, Niki didn't pay too much attention to the content. She focused on grammar, punctuation, and syntax. One paper, however, caught her attention, as it was on multiple sclerosis. One of her former college classmates had just been diagnosed. She read the paper with interest and a degree of sophistication as she had just finished the neurology module in her program. One of the conclusions didn't seem correct to her. Niki went and read some of the earlier work in this area. Niki believed the paper she was reviewing had nuanced the conclusion in the study in a way that supported the work but was not conclusively supported by the data. Niki read the paper again more carefully and again felt that the conclusions drawn were not warranted. Niki speculated whether this was accidental or deliberate and whether it was good science, inexperience, or on the edge of fraud. As a philosophical question, this interested Niki because she was considering graduate [CD1] work and a career in academics. Niki sought out the 40-year-old professor to ask whether the conclusions in the paper were appropriate and to understand the rules of the academic publishing game and the pressures that would induce a researcher to engage in such behaviors.

IV

Ryan P. really liked the department chair. Unlike most of the faculty, he had a corporate background so the two had a lot in common. After class, the chair would stay a few minutes extra and talk with Ryan. They would exchange war stories of their days in the "trenches." The chair was only 4 or 5 years older than Ryan, so they had similar taste in movies and music. Ryan decided to run a literature search to see what kind of writer and researcher the chair was. Ryan was amazed. There were over 8 to 10 publications per year for the last 8 years. The chair assumed his current position 8 years ago. Ryan noticed that none of the publications were authored only by the chair. In fact, each paper had three or four other names on it, and the titles were remarkably similar to the papers they were writing for his course. Interestingly, there were 10 groups in this year's class.

The next week after class, Ryan asked the chair about the publications and the topics for the course. The chair was perfectly candid. He said he was under the gun to publish and since he provided the framework for the papers in the class, even though he didn't write or edit any of the paper, he believed he had a right to authorship. No student had ever refused his request to have his name included on their work. Ryan realized how untenable a student's position would be if they asked to be included as author. This struck Ryan as completely unfair. He wondered what he would say if the chair asked for authorship on his group's paper.

✳ LEARNING OBJECTIVES

- Discuss the three personality traits of the dark side.
- Describe the reasons for dark side behaviors.
- List the motives for a moral outrage.
- Discuss impairment among health practitioners.

✳ KEY TERMS

- Machiavellianism
- Moral outrages
- Narcissism
- Psychopathy

The Dark Side

PROFESSIONAL STATUS CONFERS UNUSUAL POWER and autonomy on individuals within the practice of that profession. That power and autonomy can be abused. Seven behaviors—when exhibited—diminish individual professionalism, compromise care, weaken the healthcare system, and erode patient trust and confidence. Those seven behaviors, when bundled together, can be termed the dark side of professionalism. These seven behaviors are as follows (Data from American Board of Internal Medicine 2001):

- **Abuse of power:** Society confers power on individuals as professionals and typically abides by the recommendations of the professional. If this power is used for reasons other than the betterment of the patient and society, typically for personal gain, then abuse occurs. Abuse of power can occur in relationships with patients and colleagues. This abuse manifests itself in bias, sexual harassment, and breaches in confidentiality.

- **Arrogance:** Arrogance is an offensive display of superiority and self-importance resulting in haughtiness, vanity, insolence, and disdain.
- **Greed:** Greed predominates when money becomes the driving force. Greed is an inordinate pursuit of power, fame, and money.
- **Misrepresentation:** Misrepresentation is lying and fraud. Lying is consciously failing to tell the truth. Fraud is a conscious misrepresentation of fact intended to mislead.
- **Impairment:** Impairment occurs as a result of alcohol, drugs, or mental impairment.
- **Lack of conscientiousness:** Lack of conscientiousness is the failure to fulfill responsibilities.
- **Conflict of interest:** A situation where the interest of the practitioner is placed above the patient is a conflict of interest.

The Dark Side and Personal Growth

THE PSYCHOLOGIST CARL JUNG THEORIZED that we all have a "shadow self" and a "dark side." Further, according to Jung, the less we acknowledge this dark side, the blacker it is and the more sinister. The dark side of our personalities houses the evil we are capable of. Personal growth occurs in acknowledging this potential in each of us. We all have the urge sometimes to cheat, crush, or kill; it is only circumstance and our sense of right and wrong that prevent us from carrying out these urges. Innumerable classroom exercises demonstrate that each of us will gladly sacrifice one individual to save multiple others or steal to acquire a life-saving drug if no other means were available. Which of us would not go to any length to save one of our children? Before you discount the notion of a dark side, think of circumstances where you would be likely to engage in fraud or alleviate the pain of one of life's tragedies with drugs or alcohol. Access the newsletter from your state board of licensure and notice the number of licenses that get suspended for impairment or financial misdeeds. It is not likely that all of the cases reflect the behavior of psychopaths and narcissists; most were probably well-meaning professionals (once students like you) who got caught in circumstances that opened the trap door to their unacknowledged dark side. Professional, mature practitioners recognize we are all capable of "dark side" transgressions.

Is the Dark Side a Dichotomous Variable?

A DICHOTOMOUS VARIABLE IS AN EITHER–OR proposition. In most circumstances, one is either male or female. With rare exceptions, no person is either completely evil or completely good. Most of us are mosaics of both traits, good at some things and not others; improving on some things and regressing on others; and molded by circumstance and blown by the winds of convenience and expediency. No practitioner is likely to be characterized as completely nonprofessional. A practitioner who is defrauding Medicare may still be loved by patients for his or her empathy and willingness to serve. The dark side, then, is not a dichotomous variable, but a continuous variable that registers degrees of the nonprofessional behaviors and traits.

What Personality Traits Explain This Aspect of Professionalism?

THE DARK SIDE OF PROFESSIONALISM can be linked to personality, specifically three personality traits termed the *dark triad* (O'Boyle et al. 2011).

Machiavellianism: Machiavellianism rests on the following values: (1) a belief in the effectiveness of manipulative tactics for personal gain; (2) a cynical view of human nature; and (3) a moral outlook that elevates expediency over principle. Machiavellians are more likely to make ethically suspect decisions. They are more likely to cheat, lie, and betray others but do not typically engage in extreme forms of negative behavior.

Narcissism: Narcissism is characterized by an inflated view of the self and fantasies of control, admiration, and success. Most individuals possess some level of this trait. At the extremes, these traits become problematic. Narcissists may appear arrogant, self-promoting, and less likeable. When publicly censored or challenged, narcissists may react aggressively. At the extreme, narcissism is considered a clinical disorder, rather than a personality trait.

Psychopathy: Psychopathy is characterized by a lack of concern for others and the rules of society. A lack of guilt is associated with this trait. These people are characterized by likeability, glibness, and charm, although they are also callous, emotionally cold, and unsentimental. They often engage in parasitic lifestyles and use criminal behaviors to achieve their ends. They are associated with academic cheating. Like narcissism, at the extreme, psychopathy is a clinical disorder rather than a personality trait.

In short, the dark sides of professional behavior are simply expressions of inherent personality traits termed the *dark triad*. The dark triad represents a social engagement strategy based on exploitation. Each personality trait involves a high degree of selfishness and elevating one's personal needs over the needs of others. Because these traits are not socially desirable, individuals often try to hide them. Along with this external deception, there is often a high level of internal deception regarding these traits as individuals rationalize to themselves why they must engage in this pattern.

How Do You Explain These Behaviors?

THE DARK SIDE OF PROFESSIONALISM can be explained from multiple perspectives. Each offers insight into these behaviors. As with all explanations for human behavior, each of these insights is limited in some manner. Taken together, they give a reasonable explanation for this pattern of professional behavior.

- These behaviors may arise as a function of the impact of cultural norms and the economic system. A consumer focus and a ruthless Social Darwinism, unfettered by perspective, may lead to a disregard for others and a sense that "I have to get mine."
- An unconscious need felt as a constant hunger, a feeling of being alone and of being empty, may lead to selfish gratification and a ruthless pursuit of money and power.
- Schemas are theories of the self, others, and the world that serve as cognitive frames for behavior. In other words, what is believed

about the self, others, and the world drives behaviors. Inappropriate schemas reflecting abandonment, entitlement, specialness, omnipotence, perfectionism, inability to be satisfied, and so on provide templates for justifying ruthless professional actions.

- From an evolutionary perspective, behaviors have been selected for their impact on species survival and then transmitted to subsequent generations. In appropriate doses, the behavioral patterns of the dark triad can be presumed to enhance survival for the individual. In short, there is a genetic basis for the behaviors of the dark triad.
- These behaviors may simply be learned. Association with respected mentors who exhibit these behaviors may lead a novice professional to assume that these are the rules of the game for getting ahead.
- Like all behaviors, their variation can be arrayed along a bell curve. People who exhibit the dark triad are simply those at the tail of a normal distribution anchored by good at one tail and evil at the other. Deficiencies in the brain chemistry and circuitry may account for the nonprofessional behaviors. At least 10 interconnected brain regions are involved in an empathy circuit. Deficiencies in these regions explain this distribution.
- Parenting that was neglectful or abusive may lie at the root of the nonprofessional behaviors.

The interesting question is why someone who has economic security, status, and power as a result of their professional licensure would feel the need to risk it by violating the standards of the profession.

Moral Outrages

DOCTORS, NURSES, PHARMACISTS, AND OTHER healthcare professionals who consciously and overtly kill multiple patients are relatively rare but not uncommon. Yorker et al. (2006) identified 90 cases of serial murder by healthcare professionals worldwide. By far, most (86%) of the serial killers were nurses. It seems incongruent that individuals who work to become caregivers in fact set about to harm patients. Behaviors and traits of practitioners that seem to indicate suspicious activities include the following (Data from Ramsland 2012):

- Nicknames such as Dr. Death
- Entered rooms where unexpected deaths occurred

- Frequent movement from one facility to another
- Difficult personal relationships
- Liked to "predict" when a patient would die
- Made inconsistent statements following suspicious incidents
- Preferred shifts with little supervision
- Were associated with several incidents at different institutions
- Craved attention
- Complained about the burden of patients
- Kept others from checking on patients
- Were seen in areas where they did not belong
- Hung around for the immediate death investigation
- Possessed the suspected substance at home, in a locker, or in personal effects
- Lied about personal details or credentials
- Had been involved in other types of criminal activities
- Had substance abuse problems

Motives for these **moral outrages** include the following (Data from Ramsland 2007):

- The desire to be a hero. They create medical emergencies so they can play a lead role to win accolades.
- The need for attention. This is associated with a personality disorder termed *Munchausen syndrome by proxy* where one individual harms another to gain notice for themselves.
- To experiment with the human body without being discovered.
- For the thrill or excitement. The heightened feeling associated with the act is akin to a sexual encounter.
- To feel empowered or gain control.
- Necrophiliac voyeurism, the embrace of life over death, or a malignant aggression to make a destructive mark. A keen interest in sickness and death and an insensitivity to tragedy.
- To gain relief from inner conflicts and turmoil.
- A fear of a loss of control; often true of the adult children of alcoholics.
- Predatory challenge/addiction. The compulsion to beat the system.
- Poor self-esteem that manifests itself as a disdain for the patient.
- A perverted compassion to ease pain and suffering.
- To ease the workload.

- For profit.
- To make colleagues look bad.

Most serial killers are self-obsessed and convinced of their own superiority. Many are angry and believe that life is unfair. Thus, others must pay. Most serial killers are narcissistic, impulsive, and callous psychopaths. For them, it does not matter who they hurt as long as they get their way. They tend not to feel remorse and are adept at compartmentalizing and exhibiting a socially acceptable "good" self while hiding the "dark" self. They are like Dr. Jekyl and Mr. Hyde.

Fraud

HEALTH CARE IS A HUGE business in the United States, in excess of $2 trillion. It is also complex and complicated. Industry structure provides great opportunities for fraud in that there are multiple payors to multiple independent providers where the actual consumer of the products or services is disconnected from the billing and payment process, eliminating a significant control point. Estimates of fraud in the United States range from $100 to $600 billion annually (Byrd, Powell, and Smith 2013). CNN Money reports that a single physician in Dallas bilked Medicare for over $375 million over 5 years in a home healthcare scam (Kavilanz 2012).

The Association of Certified Fraud Examiners defines a fraud as a material false statement, knowledge that the statement was false, reliance on the false statement by the victim, and damages resulting from the reliance by the victim on the false statement. Actions that negatively impact the system but that occur inadvertently, without malice or intent to defraud, are not considered fraud. Examples include deficient understanding of coding rules or incomplete ethical understanding. It is intent that is the determining factor in fraud.

Types of fraud include provider frauds or false claim schemes and quality data reporting fraud involving the provision of medically unnecessary services and failure of care. This type of fraud also includes research fraud, falsified drug testing results, falsified clinical trial results, and uncertified or unlicensed providers providing and billing for care outside their scope of practice. Most fraud is discussed in financial terms but may include medication substitution, counterfeit drugs and other products, administrative corruption, discrimination in providing services, and illegal purchase and sale of transplant organs.

All healthcare fraud occurs because someone has the opportunity to commit a fraud, the motivation to do it, and a rationalization or justification for the fraud (e.g., the reimbursement is too low). These three elements constitute the "fraud triangle." Fraud may also occur based on the belief that it was necessary to preserve a human life.

Why the Dark Side?

THOSE CAPABLE OF DARK SIDE actions have a characteristic and pronounced lack of empathy, which is the ability to perceive and intuit what another person is thinking or feeling and respond to those thoughts and feelings in an inappropriate manner. A lower level of empathy is termed *affective contagion*, which is the ability at a subconscious and involuntary level to understand how another person feels. A higher order of empathy is termed *cognitive empathy*, which is a complex, conscious, and willful attempt to understand another person's internal state. Cognitive empathy includes an attempt to understand another person's motives and beliefs. It is a deficiency in empathy that explains dark side behaviors. Like all human traits, empathy is normally distributed through the population. As such, some individuals will display no empathy while others display remarkable empathy. Individuals with no empathy (level 0) are capable of murder, torture, rape, and other crimes. At this level, the fact that someone was hurt means nothing. The criminals experience no remorse or guilt. At level 1 of empathy, individuals are capable of hurting others but can reflect to some extent on the consequences. These individuals can feel for another person, but their empathy is insufficient to control their impulses. Once those impulses are engaged, another person's feelings do not matter (Baron-Cohen 2011).

Why Do People Lie?

LYING IS NOT THE EXCEPTION in human behavior. On average, people tell three lies for every 15 minutes of conversation (Bartolini 2004). Lying is often spontaneous and unconscious, devoid of cynicism. The reasons people lie include the following (Data from Williams et al. 2009):

- People lie because they like to; they derive pleasure and a sense of power from it.
- People lie to gain an advantage.

- People lie to achieve an end result.
- People lie because it is socially advantageous to them and enhances social prestige.
- People lie as a means of self-preservation, beginning with a white lie and spreading to a complex web of deceit.
- People lie to avoid punishment.
- People lie because deception is required to function in daily life.
- People lie because the truth may be hurtful, difficult, or painful.
- Excessive lying may be a warning sign and plea for help.
- People lie to protect their innermost thoughts and feelings.

Only the extremely naïve would discount the value of relatively harmless lies that smooth out and maintain the social fabric. Lies that significantly favor one party at the expense of another are a different matter. A professional who "shades" advice and recommendations to unduly profit and compromise another is clearly outside this realm of lies as social lubrication. A lie told to a child about to undergo an uncomfortable round of chemotherapy is an act of professional kindness, but a lie regarding a fatal mistake to protect a license is not.

The Impaired Practitioner

A PROFESSIONAL LICENSE TO PRACTICE CAN last a practitioner's entire life, as long as continuing education requirements are met and no substantial ethical or legal actions are taken against the practitioner. At the extreme, incompetent practitioners are disciplined via state boards and the legal system as errors and malpractice incidents accrue. This leaves considerable room for an impaired practitioner to practice, make errors, and hurt patients. The American Medical Association defines impairment as "any physical, mental, or behavioral disorder that interferes with ability to engage safely in professional activities."

Health care is a stressful activity, as is healthcare education. That practitioners and students suffer from stress, anxiety, burnout, and depression is not surprising. Psychiatric and emotional impairment can range from full-blown psychiatric disorders to situational and transient depression. It is estimated that 26.2% of Americans over 18 years old suffer from a diagnosable mental disorder in any given year. About 6% suffer from serious mental illness (Kessler et al. 2005). One study suggests that 220,000 to 286,000 nurses in this country suffer from a mental disorder (Smith and Hukill 1996). It has been reported that 19.5% of female physicians have a history of depression, and 1.5% reported a history of suicide attempts. The rate of depression mirrors that of the general population (Miller and McGowen 2000).

Many healthcare professionals have relatively unsupervised access to legal pharmaceuticals. All have access to illegal pharmaceuticals through the many illicit channels available in America. Substance abuse is a recognized health issue in the general American population. It is not surprising that healthcare professionals suffer from substance abuse. Estimates suggest that 10–20% of nurses have substance abuse problems and that 6–8% of registered nurses are impaired due to alcohol or other drugs (Griffith 1999). The estimated prevalence of substance abuse among physicians, based on self-report, is 7.9%, less than the 16% prevalence in the general population (Schorling 2009). It is likely that the rate of substance abuse among physicians mirrors that of the general population. Most physicians tend to abuse minor opioids for self-treatment and alcohol for stress.

Practitioners also may be impaired due to acute or chronic disease. Diseases such as multiple sclerosis and Parkinson disease create cognitive challenges. Lethal infections such as hepatitis C or degenerative diseases such as rheumatoid arthritis circumscribe certain practice activities. The severity of the disease, its treatability, and the nature of the professional obligations are the critical variables in this context. Age is also a source of impairment. In a study in Australia, 54% of older doctors suffered cognitive impairment. Older doctors were described as suffering "the four Ds": dementia, drugs, drink, and depression (Peisah and Wilhelm 2007).

Practitioner behavior regarding impairment can be explained from various perspectives. Certain traits such as dependency, pessimism, passivity, self-doubt, low self-esteem, feelings of inadequacy, dysphoria, excessive worry, or social anxiety may explain impairment. Excess perfectionism may lead to a hyperconscientiousness and unforgiving attitude toward oneself. Unremitting workaholic standards may be contributory, as well as difficulty in setting limits and self-denial. The culture of health care itself with its emphasis on winning may be the culprit. Finally, a sense of invincibility, of being above the normal human limitations and immune to the normal human frailties, is a painful misconception. As noted by Miller and McGowen (2000), physicians are not invincible, and by extension, no healthcare practitioner is invincible.

Healthcare professionals have a duty to deal honestly and openly with patients so as to allow them to make informed decisions regarding their care. This may put the patient in the untenable position of having to determine whether the practitioner is in fact capable of rendering effective care. This dilemma can be avoided by a practitioner recognizing his or her impairment, voluntarily submitting to treatment, and refraining from practice until the impairment is corrected. A practitioner's obligation is a difficult one to standardize and to provide guidelines on. Some are judgment calls. However, if a practitioner knowingly understands he or she can't render effective care and proceeds to anyway for financial reasons or ego defense, he or she could be argued to have slipped to the dark side. Although there may be no intent to harm as in a moral outrage, the conclusion may be the same.

Generally, larger organizations have formal programs and policies that deal with this matter, particularly related to substance abuse. Programs for cognitive and emotional impairment are not as common. The ideal circumstance is that the professional recognizes the impairment and self-reports the problem and enters treatment. Typically, discovery of impairment by the company results in a punitive response by the company. Being aware of an impaired colleague, pharmacists have to balance the right of the individual practitioner to privacy with that of the health and safety of the patient and the integrity of the healthcare system. It is no small thing to report an impaired practitioner because livelihoods, careers, reputations, and families are at stake.

How to Deal with Dark Side Professionals

IT IS NOT LIKELY AS a student that you will knowingly encounter this type of professional. The key here is knowingly. It is not likely you will have sufficient encounters to pick up on this trait. As a new graduate, however, you may have to deal with this type of practitioner. A few reminders are in order. They are as follows:

- Practitioners demonstrating this behavior pattern are likely to be very good at it. They are likely to be very subtle in their methods.

Only the most egregious examples get noted, and if infrequent, they are explained by others as an aberration.

- Dark side practitioners see others as playing specific roles in their internal psychopathic drama. Specifically, they see themselves as special while others are pawns, patrons, patsies, and police. They have the inability to be modest, to accept blame, to act predictably, to react calmly, and to act without aggression. Their goal will be to sabotage your career.

- Be cautious in labeling someone a psychopath. Although several psychopathic tendencies may be evident, only strong evidence should support this designation.

- Greater personal insight reveals personal vulnerabilities and weaknesses that dark side practitioners may prey on. Understand which of your buttons a psychopath might push. The desire to want to "save" someone else should be a red flag. Psychopaths will draw you in and try and establish a personal bond, to your detriment and to their benefit.

- If you believe you are dealing with a psychopathic boss or coworker, document your encounters and their behaviors for your file. Because these people will be adept at sullying your reputation, documentation with dates, times, and contemporaneous summaries of conversations will support your claims.

- If changing the situation is impossible, then the best option is to leave. But do so under your own terms as much as possible. Be professional. Get on with your life and career. Avoid assuming any guilt for this circumstance. Some circumstances simply cannot be overcome.

Conclusion

THIS CHAPTER INTRODUCED THE IDEA of the "dark side" of professionalism—the idea that the power and autonomy associated with the prerogatives of professionalism can be abused. The dark triad of personality traits—Machiavellianism, narcissism, and psychopathy—was discussed. Moral outrages, fraud, and impaired practitioners were also considered.

What Do the Practitioners/Others Say?

FOR NEXT CLASS, BE PREPARED to discuss the dark side of practice based on any *one* of the following:

- A discussion with your colleagues, or others, on how they feel and what they know about the dark side of practice.
- An article on the dark side, either from the research literature or any other source.
- A movie, television program, or YouTube video about the dark side.
- A book on the dark side (literary, historical, psychological, or any other source).

Personal Learning Plan: Impressions

USE THE FOLLOWING GUIDE TO develop a personal learning plan for yourself on establishing credibility.

What prompted you to develop this plan?	
What is the general area for improvement?	
What is the specific issue for improvement?	
Why is this important to you?	
How do you generally act in these areas?	
What are your goals?	
What strategies are required?	
Who/what is necessary to meet your goals with this strategy?	
How will you measure success/failure with this effort?	
How will you reflect and capture the lesson from this effort that can be generalized to other circumstances?	

The Students: Personal and Professional Issues

B ASED ON THE DESCRIPTION OF each student at the beginning of the chapter, what are the personal and professional issues (either immediately or in the future) confronting each student? Consider whether they are linked and, if so, how. Finally, what would you recommend to each student to resolve these issues?

Dana S.

Personal Issues

Professional Issues

Are They Linked? Will the Personal Issues Impact Professional Behavior?

Recommendations

Ivan T.

Personal Issues

Professional Issues

Are They Linked? Will the Personal Issues Impact Professional Behavior?

Recommendations

Niki M.

Personal Issues

Professional Issues

Are They Linked? Will the Personal Issues Impact Professional Behavior?

Recommendations

Ryan P.

Personal Issues

Professional Issues

Are They Linked? Will the Personal Issues Impact Professional Behavior?

Recommendations

Exercises

Dark Triad

1. Ask yourself whether any of the following statements are true about you.

I tend to manipulate others to get my way.

I have used deceit or lied to get my way.

I have used flattery to get my way.

I tend to exploit others toward my own end.

I tend to lack remorse.

I tend to be unconcerned with the morality of my actions.

I tend to be callous or insensitive.

I tend to be cynical.

I tend to want others to admire me.

I tend to want others to pay attention to me.

I tend to seek prestige or status.

I tend to expect special favors from others.

The more of these statements that are true about you, the greater is your tendency to have one of the "dark side" traits.

2. With two or three of your classmates, research the state licensing board policy for impaired practitioners.

3. With two or three of your classmates, determine whether your state has a program for impaired practitioners.

4. With two or three of your classmates, research the Michael Jackson and Elvis Presley cases. Comment on the behavior of the health practitioners involved.

5. Read the Robert Courtney Case and comment on his motivation.

6. Write a one-page executive summary of the chapter.

7. Review the mind map from the opening of the chapter. Would you change anything after reading the chapter?

The Robert Courtney Case

Life had been good to Robert Courtney. Born in 1952 and graduating from pharmacy school in 1975, by age 40 he owned two pharmacies in Kansas City, Missouri. He drove a Mercedes, could buy his second wife a four-carat diamond, was planning to build a 5,000 square foot house, and had pledged $1 million dollars to his church's building fund. His family described him as an ideal son. His patients loved him, describing him as a gentleman who was always fastidiously dressed and groomed.

Though a gentleman, his moods could shift from ebullience to aloofness. His second wife described how his face would harden during a disagreement and take on a crazed look like he wanted to murder someone. Once, he slapped one of his daughters at home following a public disagreement. He needed to be in control. He would often dictate his wife's attire to attend a church event.

In 2002 Courtney pled guilty to 20 federal counts of adulterating and tampering with the chemotherapy drugs Taxol and Gemzar. From 1990 to 2002, it is estimated that Courtney diluted 98,000 prescriptions for 4,200 patients involving 72 different drugs. The drugs involved were antibiotics, drugs to improve clotting, and fertility drugs. Courtney often substituted generic drugs for name brand drugs that had been specified. In addition, Courtney brought drugs through the gray market, outside the normal channels of distribution. He was sentenced to 30 years in federal prison and named as defendant in 300 suits for fraud and wrongful death. He was also hit with a judgment in the amount of $2.2 billion.

What Robert Courtney was doing, in essence, was providing sick and dying patients sterile water rather than the called for life saving drugs. In doing so, Courtney had amassed over $18 million in assets, an amount that would be impossible to earn from running two small pharmacies.

The question is: How do you explain Courtney's behavior?

Data from, Draper, R. (2003). The toxic pharmacist. *New York Times,* June 8.

What's Important to You in the Chapter?

W ITH SEVERAL OF YOUR CLASSMATES, discuss the idea or ideas that are most likely to effect a change in your values, attitudes, or behaviors. Be succinct. Write no more than two sentences.

References

American Board of Internal Medicine. (2001). Project Professionalism. http://www.abimfoundation.org/~/media/Foundation/Professionalism /Project%20professionalism.ashx?la=en

Baron-Cohen, S. (2011). *The Science of Evil*. New York, NY: Basic Books.

Bartolini, L. (2004). Why we lie: The evolutionary roots of deception and the unconscious mind. *Library Journal*. 129 (12), 114.

Byrd, J. D., Powell, P., and Smith, D. L. (2013). Health care fraud: An introduction to a major cost issue. *Journal of Accounting, Ethics, and Public Policy*. 14 (3), 521–539.

Griffith, J. (1999). Substance abuse disorders in nurses. *Nursing Forum*. 34 (4, October–December), 19–28.

Kavilanz, P. (February 29, 2012). CNN Money. http://money.cnn .com/2012/02/28/small business/medicare_fraud/

Kessler, R. C., Chiu, W. T., Demler, O., and Walters, E. E. (2005). Prevalence, severity, and comorbidity of twelve month DSM-IV disorders in the National Comorbidity Survey Replication (NCS-R). *Archives of General Psychiatry*. 62, 617–627.

Miller, M. N., and McGowen, K. R. (2000). The painful truth: Physicians are not invincible. *Southern Medical Journal*. 93 (10), 966–973.

O'Boyle, E. H., Forsyth, D. R., Banks, G. C., and McDaniel, M. A. (2011). A meta-analysis of the dark triad and work behavior: A social exchange perspective. *Journal of Applied Psychology*. October 24, 1–23.

Peisah, C., and Wilhelm, K. (2007). Physician don't heal thyself: A descriptive study of impaired older doctors. *International Psychogeriatrics*. 19 (5), 974–984.

Ramsland, K. (2007). *Inside the Minds of Healthcare Serial Killers*. Westport, CT: Praeger.

Ramsland, K. (2012). When nurses kill. *Psychology Today.* https://www
.psychologytoday.com/blog/shadow-boxing/201204/when-nurses-kill

Schorling, J. B. (2009). Physician impairment due to substance use disorders. www.medscape.com/viewarticle/

Smith, G. B., and Hukill, E. (1996). Nurses impaired by emotional and psychological dysfunction. *Journal of the American Psychiatric Nurses
Association.* 2 (6), 192–201.

Williams, K. C., Hernandez, E. H., Petrosky, A. R., and Page, R. A. (2009).
The business of lying. *Journal of Leadership, Accountability, and Ethics.*
Winter, 1–20.

Yorker, B. C., Kizer, K. W., Lampe, P., Forrest, A. R. W., Lannan, J. M., and
Russell, D. A. (2006). Serial murder by healthcare professionals. *Journal
of Forensic Science.* 51 (6), 1362–1371.

Suggested Readings

Austin, E. J., Farrelly, D., Black, C., and Moore, H. (2007). Emotional intelligence, Machiavellianism and emotional manipulation: Does EI have a
dark side? *Personality and Individual Differences.* 43, 179–189.

Babiak, P., and Hare, R. D. (2006). *Snakes in Suits.* New York, NY: Harper
Collins.

Brook, M., and Kosson, D. S. (2012). Impaired cognitive empathy in criminal psychopathy: Evidence from a laboratory measure of empathic
accuracy. *Journal of Abnormal Psychology.* 122 (1), 156–166.

Farber, N. J., Gilibert, S. G., Aboff, B. M., Collier, V. U., Weiner, J., and Boyer,
G. (2005). Physicians' willingness to report impaired colleagues. *Social
Science and Medicine.* 61, 1772–1775.

Gilbert, P. (2002). Evolutionary approaches to psychopathy and cognitive therapy. *Journal of Cognitive Psychotherapy: An International
Quarterly.* 16 (3), 263–294.

Jonason, P. K., and Webster, G. D. (2010). The dirty dozen: A concise measure of the dark triad. *Psychological Assessment.* 22 (2), 420–432.

Kenna, G. A., Erickson, C., and Tommasello, A. (2006). Understanding
substance abuse and dependence by the pharmacy profession. *U. S.
Pharmacist.* 5, 21–33.

Leahy, R. L. (1992). Cognitive therapy on Wall Street: Schemas and scripts of invulnerability. *Journal of Cognitive Psychotherapy: An International Quarterly*. 6 (4), 245–258.

Lubit, R. H. (2004). *Coping with Toxic Managers, Subordinates and Other Difficult People*. Upper Saddle River, NJ: FT Press.

Maher, B. A., and Maher, W. B. (1994). Personality and psychopathology: A historical perspective. *Journal of Abnormal Psychology*. 103 (1), 72–77.

Nikelly, A. (2006). The pathogenesis of greed: Causes and consequences. *International Journal of Applied Psychoanalytic Studies*. 3 (1), 65–78.

Perper, J. A., and Cina, S. J. (2010). *When Doctors Kill*. New York, NY: Copernicus Books.

Reimann, M., and Zimbardo, P. G. (2014). The dark side of social encounters: Prospects for a neuroscience of human evil. *Journal of Neuroscience, Psychology, and Economics*. 4 (3), 174–180.

Sparrow, M. K. (2000). *License to Steal*. Boulder, CO: Westview Press.

Waska, R. (2004). Greed and the frightening rumble of psychic hunger. *The American Journal of Psychoanalysis*. 64 (3), 253–266.

CHAPTER 5

Personality

Preassessment: Personality

Mind Mapping

Consider the phrase displayed on the page. For this phrase, without thinking or editing, write down the ideas, concepts, examples, contradictions, and theories that come to mind. Do not array them in any systematic or orderly manner. Scatter them about the page. Now, draw lines between your additions, indicating that there is a relationship between the terms. If something causes something else, indicate this with an arrow. Relationships may be reciprocal, meaning both cause each other, requiring arrows at both ends. Indicate the strength of the relationships by darkening and thickening the lines; stronger relationships have darker and thicker lines. **Most important: There is no right answer. Do not compare with your classmates.** *What you have is a mind map, your mental representation of these topics. Review to determine if anything has changed following this section.*

You

(What comes to mind when you think of yourself?)

The Students

I

SAYING WHAT SHE FELT WAS liberating. It felt good. Dana S. practiced it first with her mother. Each time her mother excessively intruded or tried to micromanage her life, Dana spoke up. She was nice about it, but she let her mother know that her input was not appreciated, especially when it wasn't asked for or was condescending. Surprisingly, it seemed there was a newfound respect from her mother. She had started practicing the same responses with the technicians at work. It seemed to be going well. She planned to move on to her colleagues next and ultimately to her superiors. The last rung would be challenging, as Dana always had an inordinate fear of authority. Dana noticed that each time she asserted herself, it was on a day when things were going well and she felt good about herself.

Lately, the weather had been miserable. Four days of thunderstorms were followed by overcast skies and high humidity. It was so muggy that Dana started to sweat on her walk to the car. Dana never sweat. She was rail thin with almost no body fat. She generally wore a sweater at work, as she was always cold. The excessive rains had caused her garage to fill up with water as the drains couldn't accommodate the run off. Sitting at the stoplight, she opened her mail. She had just gotten an overdraft charge from the bank on her account. Dana hated this. As soon as she walked in the door, Dana noticed the air conditioner was off and the place smelled like her dog. She went to feed the dog and was out of dog food. Jumping in her car to go buy more food, she pulled out and nicked the fender of her neighbor's car. As she walked up to the door to tell the neighbor about the accident, Dana felt herself retreating into her shell.

II

Ivan T. liked talking to the old man. He was in his 80s now and had lived a rich life. He told Ivan tales of being on the road as an investment salesman back in the 1950s and traveling through small midwestern towns. The old man was full of jokes and stories. Each time he told a story, it changed. He told Ivan, "Never let the truth get in the way of a good story." Ivan could see why the man had been successful, he genuinely liked people and never seemed to get too stressed by anything. His line was, "If nobody died and no souls were lost, then it's not a problem, just fix it."

Ivan thought he had some of the same traits as the old man; one was the gift of gab and the ability to talk to anyone. When he first met someone, Ivan was charming and focused on the other person. As he got to know the person, Ivan's conversation began to become more argumentative. Ivan liked these conversations; it was just about ideas. He loved talking politics and current events. Sometimes Ivan thought he went too far. At one party, it was clear he had. The woman he was talking to said, "Look, you don't know me well enough to be this mean to me." She got up and left.

The next time Ivan met with the old man, he asked him about this. The old man told Ivan that sometimes Ivan was like putting on a suit that was itchy, that he took some time to get used to. Ivan left contemplating what this meant, what he really felt about people, and what he was willing to do to get along others.

III

Niki M. loved this time of year. She lived in a great neighborhood. The kids walked to and from school every day. Sometimes before taking her son to kindergarten, she would sit and watch the kids go by. Two little boys would come by and stop and talk to her. One had red hair, and the other always wore a Michael Jordan sweatband. They must have been in second grade.

Now that she was finished with school, Niki had more time to spend with her mother and father. She actually spent more time with them now, even though she had moved across town, than when she lived in their basement. She had always had a somewhat distant relationship with her mother. Niki felt that her mother always liked her older brother better. Niki thought her desire to succeed and her competitiveness (some say hypercompetitiveness) were somehow linked to these feelings. She remembered ice cream night when they were children. She was still convinced that her mother gave her brother more ice cream than she got. When she thought about it, Niki realized that her mother did not have female friends. All the men seemed to congregate around her mother at parties. She seemed to generally like male-dominated conversation, and the men seemed to appreciate her willingness to give and take. She knew her mother doted on her father. When she was young and he returned from a business trip, she and her brother were shunted to their rooms.

Now, her son was bringing Niki and her mother closer together. They discussed child rearing and often times from her own childhood. She asked her mother about her relationship with her father. Niki never knew this, but her mother said she had almost left him a year after they were married. Her mother said she packed her bags one day, waited for Niki's father to return, and told him that unless he changed his obsessive control over the details of their life she was leaving. Niki wanted to hear more about this.

IV

Ryan P. had always been easy going. He took things in stride. If there was a problem, he didn't worry about it; he just fixed it and moved on. He sensed school was changing him. He was tense all the time. The stack of notes he was forced to memorize seemed to grow with each class. It was a constant day-to-day attention to his work that kept him in the program. There never seemed to be any down time. Small things bothered him now. Generally, he viewed his daughters' rooms as their private domain. Each time he walked past them now, he would get angrier and angrier. Last Sunday night after returning from class, he lashed out at his youngest daughter about her room. He even began to be critical of his wife's efforts in the house. He was irked the other day that his socks weren't matched properly. The stress of going to school, borrowing money for tuition, and living on a reduced income strained his relationship with his wife.

If school stressed Ryan out this much, what would practice do, with the pressure of not making a mistake? Ryan knew that experiences changed people, and he wondered if he would be the same when he graduated.

⚙ LEARNING OBJECTIVES

- Discuss the big five personality traits.
- Discuss the link between personality and the core values of professionalism.
- Discuss the link between personality and the psychology of professionalism.
- Discuss whether personality can change.

✤ KEY TERMS

- Agreeableness
- Conscientiousness
- Extraversion
- Neuroticism
- Openness to experience
- Personality

What Is Personality?

WHEN YOU ASK YOURSELF, "WHO am I?" or "What makes me who I am?" you are really asking what about your **personality**. Personality is a relatively enduring pattern of thoughts, feelings, and behaviors that distinguish individuals from one another. Personality development emerges early in life and continues to develop over the life span. It has been shown that as much as 50% of the variation in personality may be attributed to genetics, suggesting, for example, that the tendency toward depression may have a genetic basis. However, the environment can moderate that tendency. Children raised by a depressive parent may not become depressed contingent on what happens in their life. Life's experiences may reinforce certain genetic tendencies or ameliorate them. This explains why children raised in the same family develop different personalities. The historian Barbara Tuchman (1981, p. 255) describes it this way: "In combination of personality, circumstance, and historical moment, each man is a package of variables impossible to duplicate. His birth, his parents, his siblings, his food, his home, his school, his economic and social status, his first job, his first girl, and the variables inherent in all of these, make up that mysterious compendium, personality." There are as many personalities as there are people on the planet. In thinking about personality, it is helpful to remember that each person is:

Like all other people,

Like some other people, and

Like no other people (Kluckhohn and Murray 1953, p. 53).

The Big Five

HISTORICALLY, THERE HAVE BEEN DIFFERING views on personality: psychodynamic—the struggle between animal instinct and the pressures of socialization; traits—people exhibit consistent psychological traits; humanistic—people seek personal growth and fulfillment; and social cognitive—people behave according to how they cope with social pressure and solve social problems. Although there are as many personalities as there are people on the planet, we are all alike at some level. In fact, we are more alike than different. That similarity is captured in the dominant view of personality today—the "Big Five" theory of personality. This theory suggests that all personality variables and traits can be collapsed into the following five factors: conscientiousness, agreeableness, neuroticism, openness to experience, and extraversion (CANOE).

Conscientiousness

THE TRAIT RELATED TO IMPULSE control is called **conscientiousness**. People who score high in this trait are disciplined, organized, goal driven, and self-controlled compared with low scorers who are impulsive and spontaneous. Occupational success is more closely related to the trait of conscientiousness than other traits. Those high in conscientiousness are described as perfectionists and workaholics, and often people who score high in this trait find it difficult to be flexible when adjusting to a change of routine. People who score high in this trait are often perceived as being intelligent and dependable. Those who score high in conscientiousness are described as always prepared, liking order, following a schedule, paying attention to details, and getting work done right away. Six useful subscales are associated with conscientiousness:

- Self-efficacy—taking pride in your work, performing in a competent fashion
- Orderliness—neat, tidy, scheduled
- Dutifulness—related to job delinquency, substance abuse
- Achievement striving—the desire to move up

- Self-discipline—the ability to keep working
- Cautiousness—related to impulsive behavior

Agreeableness

AGREEABLENESS IS A TRAIT THAT is related to empathy and understanding. Individuals who score high in this trait are often described as being cooperative, trusting, and empathic in contrast to low scorers who can be described as cold, hostile, and noncooperative. Paying attention to the mental states of others, helping others, and having good interpersonal relationships are traits of someone who scores high in agreeableness. Research in personality has discovered that women score higher in agreeableness than men. Those who score high in agreeableness are described as being interested in people, being aware of others' emotions, having a soft heart, taking time for others, and being sympathetic to others' feelings. Subscales related to agreeableness include:

- Trust—believing the best about people
- Morality—a strong sense of right and wrong
- Altruism—the desire to help others
- Cooperation—wanting to get along
- Modesty—not thinking of oneself as special
- Sympathy—concern for others

Neuroticism

INDIVIDUALS WHO SCORE HIGH IN **neuroticism** tend to be anxious, insecure, and prone to stress and worry and are more affected by the daily hassles of life than low scorers. Neuroticism has been described as the response to negative emotions. Examples of negative emotions include fear, anxiety, shame, guilt, disgust, and sadness. Neuroticism has been related to depression, anxiety disorders, phobia, eating disorders, posttraumatic stress disorder, and obsessive-compulsive disorder. People who score on the high end of neuroticism often have low self-esteem and are constantly wondering if they have taken the right path in life. Self-doubt is a common theme. People on the low end of neuroticism tend to be calm and display emotional stability. Individuals with high levels of neuroticism could be described as easily disturbed, easily irritated, easily stressed, prone to frequent mood swings, and engaged in excessive worry. The subscales related to neuroticism are:

- Anxiety—nervousness, unease
- Anger—annoyance, displeasure, hostility
- Depression—despondency, hopelessness, inadequacy
- Self-consciousness—social anxiety, unassertive
- Immoderation—poor impulse control
- Vulnerability—easily flustered, difficulty in performing under stress

Openness to Experience

THE TRAIT OF OPENNESS TO experience refers to those individuals who are creative and imaginative and prefer variety over routine. High scorers are open to experience, are intellectually curious, have an appreciation for art, and are aware of their feelings. They like uniqueness. A high scorer in openness to experience would be full of ideas, quick to understand things, have a vivid imagination, spend time reflecting on things, and have a rich vocabulary. The subscales related to openness to experience include:

- Imagination—creative, can get lost in their thoughts
- Artistic interests—interest in music, art, and so on
- Emotionality—experience and express emotions
- Adventurousness—love of the new and different
- Intellect—high value on intellectual pursuits
- Liberalism—support for the liberal perspective

Extraversion

CARL JUNG INTRODUCED THE TERMS extroversion and introversion in 1921. His idea of an extrovert was someone who was focused outward, liked action more than reflection, enjoyed other people's company, and was outgoing and active. In contrast, the introvert was described as someone who is in tune with his own thoughts and feelings, seeks solitude to reflect, and is aloof and quiet. The core of extroversion is sociability. Extroverts tend to be ambitious, enjoy gaining status and receiving social attention, and have lots of positive emotion in their daily lives. Individuals who score high in extroversion report more states of joy, desire, enthusiasm, and excitement than low scorers (i.e., positive emotions). Someone high in extraversion would be described as comfortable around people, the life of the party, starting conversations, and being the center of attention. The subscales linked to extraversion include:

- Friendliness—kind and pleasant
- Gregariousness—sociable, fond of company
- Assertiveness—socially appropriate expression of thoughts and feelings
- Activity level—doers
- Excitement seeking—trying new things, taking a calculated risk
- Cheerfulness—happy, optimistic

Does Personality Change?

ONE QUESTION IS WHETHER PERSONALITY is stable or whether it changes. The answer is that personality does change. It would be convenient if there were absolutes with regard to this question. For example, conscientiousness would always increase with age, regardless of what happens in a person's life. Unfortunately, this is not possible. It is possible to make some statements about personality change, although not unequivocally. When comparing a teacher assessment of school children with a subsequent interview and assessment of the same people over 40 years later, the finding was that the individuals were "recognizably the same person" (Nave et al. 2010, p. 8). People and personalities change as people mature. For example, conscientiousness and agreeableness may increase with age, whereas openness to experience may increase through early adulthood but decline with age. Meaningful life events, first job, marriage, birth of a child, unemployment, and other events may cause personality to change. The point is that personality does change. At the genetic, biochemical, and neuroscience levels, personal genetics argues for personality stability, whereas the findings on brain plasticity support personality change. To reiterate, personality does change.

Personality, Fit, and Personal and Professional Growth

P ERSONALITY HAS BEEN SHOWN TO be a significant predictor of academic performance, career success, and career satisfaction. Critical to this relationship is the idea of "fit." This idea suggests that success and satisfaction are a function of the congruence between an individual's personality and the job requirements, that the choice of a profession is an expression of personality, that individuals in a profession will share similar developmental histories, and that members of a profession will share similar personality characteristics and respond to situations in a similar fashion. This idea of fit has implications for personal and professional growth. A central idea of this book is that you cannot separate the individual from his or her professional obligations and behavior. Students have to wrestle with where and how they will "fit" within the profession. Some will fit on the front line, empathically and effectively engaged with the patient; others will fit at an analytical, corporate level; some will be comforted by the structure of routine, others deadened by it. In other words, by personality, some people are artists; others are engineers. The first step in personal and professional growth is finding "fit."

Personal Intelligence

I F FIT (THE CONGRUENCE BETWEEN personality and environmental demands) is critical to career success, performance, and personal and professional growth, then the idea of personal intelligence is helpful. Personal intelligence is the "capacity to reason about personality and to use personality and personal information to enhance one's thoughts, plans, and life experience" (Mayer 2007–2008, p. 210). "Personal intelligence involves the abilities: (a) to recognize personally relevant information from introspection and from observing oneself and others, (b) to form that information into accurate models of personality, (c) to guide one's choices by using personality information where relevant, and (d) to systemize one's goals, plans, and life stories for good outcome" (Mayer 2007–2008, p. 215). Individuals learn about themselves and their personality from introspection (eavesdropping on one's feelings and thoughts and paying attention to one's inner world), self-observation (paying attention to our external acts and drawing conclusions from them as to who we are), information from informants (information gleaned from others about ourselves), and paying attention to others and their general personality traits and the link between personality traits and their expression in the world. This process lets individuals understand that certain personality traits, those they possess and that others possess, are predictive of getting along with others, being liked, being accepted, being respected, and so on.

Personality and Professionalism

UNDERSTANDING OUR OWN PERSONALITY AND some general ideas about personality allow us to make predictions. For example, a naturally gregarious individual will have a better chance at sales than an introvert. Personality predicts academic and career success and satisfaction; it can also predict professional behavior. Examine the table below. It presents the "Big Five" traits of personality, the model of professionalism, and the aspects of the psychology of professionalism.

Personality	Professionalism Model	Psychology of Professionalism
Conscientiousness	Accountability	Sensitivity
Agreeableness	Altruism	Motivation
Neuroticism	Duty, honor, integrity	Judgment
Open to experience	Excellence	Implementation
Extraversion	Respect for others	

Remember that the "Big Five" personality model has six subscales associated with each factor. It is not hard to believe that a more conscientious individual is more likely to do his or her duty or be accountable following an error or that someone high in agreeableness will be better at implementing professional judgment. The potential linkages and relationships are exhausting. Reviewing academic findings on the nuances of these relationships is tedious. We leave it to the student to accept these linkages and relationships based on their "face" validity that common sense confirms them.

Conclusion

THIS CHAPTER PROVIDED A DEFINITION of personality as a relatively fixed pattern of feelings, beliefs, and emotions that defines who we are. It introduces and describes the "Big Five" model of personality: conscientiousness, agreeable, neuroticism, openness to experience, and extraversion. It asks you to consider whether personality is stable or changes and concludes that the answer is that personality does change. The chapter also asks you to consider the idea that certain personality types may tend to behave more professionally.

What Do the Practitioners/Others Say?

FOR NEXT CLASS, BE PREPARED to discuss any of the topics on personality based on any *one* of the following:

- A discussion with your colleagues, or others, about whether they are aware of their personality and whether their personality has changed with time.
- An article on any of the big five personality traits, either from the research literature or any other source.
- A video clip on any of the big five personality traits.
- A book on personality (literary, historical, psychological, or any other source).

Personal Learning Plan: Personality

USE THE FOLLOWING GUIDE TO develop a personal learning plan for yourself to improve your understanding of your personality.

What prompted you to develop this plan?	
What is the general area for improvement?	
What is the specific issue for improvement?	
Why is this important to you?	
How do you generally act in these areas?	
What are your goals?	
What strategies are required?	
Who/what is necessary to meet your goals with this strategy?	
How will you measure success/failure with this effort?	
How will you reflect and capture the lesson from this effort that can be generalized to other circumstances?	

The Students: Personal and Professional Issues

BASED ON THE DESCRIPTION OF each student at the beginning of the chapter, what are the personal and professional issues (either immediately or in the future) confronting each student? Consider whether they are linked and, if so, how. Finally, what would you recommend to each student to resolve these issues?

Dana S.

Personal Issues

Professional Issues

Are They Linked? Will the Personal Issues Impact Professional Behavior?

Recommendations

Ivan T.

Personal Issues

Professional Issues

Are They Linked? Will the Personal Issues Impact Professional Behavior?

Recommendations

Niki M.

Personal Issues

Professional Issues

Are They Linked? Will the Personal Issues Impact Professional Behavior?

Recommendations

Ryan P.

Personal Issues

Professional Issues

Are They Linked? Will the Personal Issues Impact Professional Behavior?

Recommendations

Exercises

Professionalism Self-Assessment

Please assess yourself on the following professionalism dimensions.

Accountability									
Deficient				Adequate				Outstanding	
1	2	3	4	5	6	7	8	9	10
Altruism									
Deficient				Adequate				Outstanding	
1	2	3	4	5	6	7	8	9	10
Duty									
Deficient				Adequate				Outstanding	
1	2	3	4	5	6	7	8	9	10
Honor									
Deficient				Adequate				Outstanding	
1	2	3	4	5	6	7	8	9	10
Integrity									
Deficient				Adequate				Outstanding	
1	2	3	4	5	6	7	8	9	10
Excellence									
Deficient				Adequate				Outstanding	
1	2	3	4	5	6	7	8	9	10
Respect for Others									
Deficient				Adequate				Outstanding	
1	2	3	4	5	6	7	8	9	10

Personality Self-Assessment

Please assess yourself on the following personality dimensions. Describe yourself honestly as you are, not as you wish to be. Describe yourself in relation to others of the same age and gender.

Each scale has six subscales. When scoring the results, items marked with an (*) are reversed scored. Scores for each subscale allow you to compare your results to the population as a whole as a percentile.

The Agreeableness Scale

_____ 1. I trust others.

_____ 2. I obstruct others' plans.

_____ 3. I make people feel welcome.

_____ 4. I am easy to satisfy.

_____ 5. I make myself the center of attention.

_____ 6. I can't stand weak people.

_____ 7. I believe that people are essentially evil.

_____ 8. I would never cheat on my taxes.

_____ 9. I take no time for others.

_____ 10. I can't stand confrontations.

_____ 11. I dislike being the center of attention.

_____ 12. I sympathize with the homeless.

_____ 13. I am wary of others.

_____ 14. I stick to the rules.

_____ 15. I anticipate the needs of others.

_____ 16. I hate to seem pushy.

_____ 17. I dislike talking about myself.

_____ 18. I feel sympathy for those who are worse off than myself.

_____ 19. I suspect hidden motives in others.

_____ 20. I take advantage of others.

_____ 21. I love to help others.

_____ 22. I have a sharp tongue.

_____ 23. I boast about my virtues.

_____ 24. I value cooperation over competition.

_____ 25. I believe that others have good intentions.

_____ 26. I use flattery to get ahead.

_____ 27. I am concerned about others.

_____ 28. I contradict others.

_____ 29. I consider myself an average person.

_____ 30. I suffer from others' sorrows.

_____ 31. I trust what people say.

_____ 32. I use others for my own ends.

_____ 33. I have a good word for everyone.

_____ 34. I love a good fight.

_____ 35. I seldom toot my own horn.

_____ 36. I am not interested in other people's problems.

_____ 37. I believe that people are basically moral.

_____ 38. I know how to get around the rules.

_____ 39. I look down on others.

_____ 40. I yell at people.

_____ 41. I believe that I am better than others.

_____ 42. I tend to dislike soft-hearted people.

_____ 43. I believe in human goodness.

_____ 44. I cheat to get ahead.

_____ 45. I am indifferent to the feelings of others.

_____ 46. I insult people.

_____ 47. I think highly of myself.

_____ 48. I believe in an eye for an eye.

_____ 49. I think that all will be well.

_____ 50. I put people under pressure.

_____ 51. I make people feel uncomfortable.

_____ 52. I get back at others.

_____ 53. I have a high opinion of myself.

_____ 54. I try not to think about the needy.

_____ 55. I distrust people.

_____ 56. I pretend to be concerned for others.

_____ 57. I turn my back on others.

_____ 58. I hold a grudge.

_____ 59. I know the answers to many questions.

_____ 60. I believe people should fend for themselves.

Trust (Tr):	1, 7*, 13*, 19*, 25, 31, 37, 43, 49, 55*
Morality (Mr):	2*, 8, 14, 20*, 26*, 32*, 38*, 44*, 50*, 56*
Altruism (Al):	3, 9*, 15, 21, 27, 33, 39*, 45*, 51, 57*
Cooperation (Co):	4, 10, 16, 22*, 28*, 34*, 40*, 46*, 52*, 58*
Modesty (Md):	5*, 11, 17, 23*, 29, 35, 41*, 47*, 53*, 59*
Sympathy (Sy):	6*, 12, 18, 24, 30, 36*, 42*, 48*, 54*, 60*

NORMS

Tr	Mr	Al	Co	Md	Sy	TOTAL	PERCENTILE
43	42	45	43	37	40	250	85
38	38	41	38	32	35	221	70
33	33	36	33	26	30	191	50
28	28	31	28	20	25	161	30
23	24	27	23	15	20	132	15

The Extroversion Scale

_____ 1. I keep others at a distance.

_____ 2. I seek quiet.

_____ 3. I take charge.

_____ 4. I am always busy.

_____ 5. I love excitement.

_____ 6. I seldom joke around.

_____ 7. I warm up quickly to others.

_____ 8. I talk to a lot of different people at parties.

_____ 9. I hold back my opinions.

_____ 10. I am always on the go.

_____ 11. I dislike loud music.

_____ 12. I have a lot of fun.

_____ 13. I feel comfortable around people.

_____ 14. I enjoy being part of a group.

_____ 15. I can talk others into doing things.

_____ 16. I do a lot in my spare time.

_____ 17. I would never go hang gliding or bungee jumping.

_____ 18. I express childlike joy.

_____ 19. I act comfortably with others.

_____ 20. I involve others in what I am doing.

_____ 21. I seek to influence others.

_____ 22. I react slowly.

_____ 23. I seek adventure.

_____ 24. I radiate joy.

_____ 25. I make friends easy.

_____ 26. I love large parties.

_____ 27. I try to lead others.

_____ 28. I let things proceed at their own pace.

_____ 29. I love action.

_____ 30. I am not easily amused.

_____ 31. I cheer people up.

_____ 32. I avoid crowds.

_____ 33. I don't like to draw attention to myself.

_____ 34. I can manage many things at the same time.

_____ 35. I enjoy being part of a loud crowd.

_____ 36. I laugh my way through life.

_____ 37. I am hard to get to know.

_____ 38. I don't like crowded events.

_____ 39. I take control of things.

_____ 40. I like a leisurely lifestyle.

_____ 41. I enjoy being reckless.

_____ 42. I love life.

_____ 43. I often feel uncomfortable around others.

_____ 44. I love surprise parties.

_____ 45. I wait for others to lead the way.

_____ 46. I react quickly.

_____ 47. I act wild and crazy.

_____ 48. I look at the bright side of life.

_____ 49. I avoid contact with others.

_____ 50. I prefer to be alone.

_____ 51. I keep in the background.

_____ 52. I like to take it easy.

_____ 53. I am willing to try anything once.

_____ 54. I laugh aloud.

_____ 55. I am not really interested in others.

_____ 56. I want to be left alone.

_____ 57. I have little to say.

_____ 58. I like to take my time.

_____ 59. I seek danger.

_____ 60. I amuse my friends.

Friendliness (Fr):	1*, 7, 13, 19, 25, 31, 37*, 43*, 49*, 55*
Gregariousness (Gr):	2*, 8, 14, 20, 26, 32*, 38*, 44, 50*, 56*
Assertiveness (As):	3, 9*, 15, 21, 27, 33*, 39, 45*, 51*, 57*
Activity Level (Al):	4, 10, 16, 22*, 28*, 34, 40*, 46, 52*, 58*
Excitement Seeking (Es):	5, 11*, 17*, 23, 29, 35, 41, 47, 53, 59
Cheerfulness (Ch):	6*, 12, 18, 24, 30*, 36, 42, 48

NORMS

Fr	Gr	As	Al	Es	Ch	TOTAL	PERCENTILE
42	36	38	36	35	40	218	85
37	30	33	31	30	36	192	70
32	24	28	26	24	31	165	50
27	18	23	21	18	26	138	30
22	12	18	16	13	22	112	15

The Neuroticism Scale

_____ 1. I worry about things

_____ 2. I rarely complain.

_____ 3. I am very pleased with myself.

_____ 4. I am easily intimidated.

_____ 5. I never splurge.

_____ 6. I panic easily.

_____ 7. I adapt easily to new situations.

_____ 8. I get angry easily.

_____ 9. I often feel blue.

_____ 10. I am able to stand up for myself.

_____ 11. I often eat too much.

_____ 12. I am calm even in tense situations.

_____ 13. I don't worry about things that have already happened.

_____ 14. I get irritated easily.

_____ 15. I dislike myself.

_____ 16. I am not bothered by difficult social situations.

_____ 17. I never spend more than I can afford.

_____ 18. I become overwhelmed by events.

_____ 19. I fear for the worst.

_____ 20. I get upset easily.

_____ 21. I feel comfortable with myself.

_____ 22. I am afraid that I will do the wrong thing.

_____ 23. I am able to control my cravings.

_____ 24. I readily overcome setbacks.

_____ 25. I am afraid of many things.

_____ 26. I keep my cool.

_____ 27. I am often down in the dumps.

_____ 28. I find it difficult to approach others.

_____ 29. I don't know why I do some of the things I do.

_____ 30. I know how to cope.

_____ 31. I am not easily disturbed by events.

_____ 32. I am often in a bad mood.

_____ 33. I have a low opinion of myself.

_____ 34. I am afraid to draw attention to myself.

_____ 35. I do things that I later regret.

_____ 36. I can handle complex problems.

_____ 37. I get stressed out easily.

_____ 38. I am not easily annoyed.

_____ 39. I have frequent mood swings.

_____ 40. I am comfortable in unfamiliar situations

_____ 41. I easily resist temptations.

_____ 42. I remain calm under pressure.

_____ 43. I get caught up in my problems.

_____ 44. I seldom get mad.

_____ 45. I seldom feel blue.

_____ 46. I only feel comfortable with friends.

_____ 47. I rarely overindulge.

_____ 48. I feel that I'm unable to deal with things.

_____ 49. I am not easily bothered by things.

_____ 50. I rarely get irritated.

_____ 51. I feel that my life lacks direction.

_____ 52. I stumble over my words.

_____ 53. I go on binges.

_____ 54. I can't make up my mind.

_____ 55. I am relaxed most of the time.

_____ 56. I lose my temper.

_____ 57. I feel desperate.

_____ 58. I am not embarrassed easily.

_____ 59. I love to eat.

_____ 60. I get overwhelmed by emotions.

Anxiety (Ax):   1, 7*, 13* 19, 25, 31*, 37, 43, 49*, 55*

Anger (Ar):   2*, 8, 14, 20, 26*, 32, 38*, 44*, 50*, 56

Depression (De):   3*, 9, 15, 21*, 27, 33, 39, 45*, 51, 57

Self-Consciousness (Sc):   4*, 10, 16*, 22, 28, 34, 40*, 46, 52, 58*

Immoderation (Im):   5*, 11, 17*, 23*, 29, 35, 41*, 47*, 53, 59

Vulnerability (Vu):   6, 12*, 18, 24*, 30*, 36*, 42*, 48, 54, 60

NORMS

Ax	Ar	De	Sc	Im	Vu	TOTAL	PERCENTILE
32	30	29	33	34	27	186	85
27	25	24	28	29	22	154	70
21	19	18	22	23	17	121	50
15	13	13	16	17	12	88	30
10	10	10	11	12	10	60	15

The Openness to Experience Scale

_____ 1. I have a vivid imagination.

_____ 2. I do not enjoy watching dance performances.

_____ 3. I don't understand people who get emotional.

_____ 4. I am attached to conventional ways.

_____ 5. I avoid difficult reading material.

_____ 6. I like to stand during the national anthem.

_____ 7. I have difficulty imagining things.

_____ 8. I believe in the importance of art.

_____ 9. I experience very few emotional highs and lows.

_____ 10. I prefer variety to routine.

_____ 11. I like to solve complex problems.

_____ 12. I believe that we should be tough on crime.

_____ 13. I enjoy wild flights of fantasy.

_____ 14. I like music.

_____ 15. I rarely notice my emotional reactions.

_____ 16. I like to visit new places.

_____ 17. I love to read challenging material.

_____ 18. I tend to vote for liberal political candidates.

_____ 19. I love to daydream.

_____ 20. I see beauty in things that others might not notice.

_____ 21. I experience my emotions intensely.

_____ 22. I am interested in many things.

_____ 23. I have a rich vocabulary.

_____ 24. I believe that there is no absolute right or wrong.

_____ 25. I seldom get lost in thought.

_____ 26. I do not like concerts.

_____ 27. I am not easily affected by my emotions.

_____ 28. I dislike new foods.

_____ 29. I am not interested in theoretical discussions.

_____ 30. I believe that we coddle criminals too much.

_____ 31. I do not have a good imagination.

_____ 32. I do not enjoy going to art museums.

_____ 33. I seldom get emotional.

_____ 34. I am a creature of habit.

_____ 35. I can handle a lot of information.

_____ 36. I believe that criminals should receive help rather than punishment.

_____ 37. I like to get lost in thought.

_____ 38. I love flowers.

_____ 39. I feel others' emotions.

_____ 40. I don't like the idea of change.

_____ 41. I have difficulty understanding abstract ideas.

_____ 42. I believe laws should be strictly enforced.

_____ 43. I seldom daydream.

_____ 44. I do not like poetry.

_____ 45. I am passionate about causes.

_____ 46. I like to begin new things.

_____ 47. I avoid philosophical discussions.

_____ 48. I believe that too much tax money goes to support artists.

_____ 49. I indulge in my fantasies.

_____ 50. I enjoy the beauty of nature.

_____ 51. I enjoy examining myself and my life.

_____ 52. I prefer to stick with things that I know.

_____ 53. I enjoy thinking about things.

_____ 54. I believe in one true religion.

_____ 55. I spend time reflecting on things.

_____ 56. I do not like art.

_____ 57. I try to understand myself.

_____ 58. I dislike changes.

_____ 59. I am not interested in abstract ideas.

_____ 60. I tend to vote for conservative political candidates.

Imagination (Im):	1, 7*, 13, 19, 25*, 31*, 37, 43*, 49, 55
Artistic Interests (Ai):	2*, 8, 14, 20, 26*, 32*, 38, 44*, 50, 56*
Emotionality (Em):	3*, 9*, 15*, 21, 27*, 33*, 39, 45, 51, 57
Adventurousness (Ad):	4*, 10, 16, 22, 28*, 34*, 40*, 46, 52*, 58
Intellect (In):	5*, 11, 17, 23, 29*, 35, 41*, 47*, 53, 59*
Liberalism (Li):	6*, 12*, 18, 24, 30*, 36, 42*, 48*, 54*, 60*

NORMS

Im	Ai	Em	Ad	In	Li	TOTAL	PERCENTILE
41	46	42	39	42	32	240	85
36	41	37	34	37	26	208	70
30	36	31	29	31	19	175	50
24	31	25	24	25	12	142	30
19	26	20	19	20	10	110	15

The Conscientiousness Scale

_____ 1. I complete tasks successfully.

_____ 2. I am bothered by disorder.

_____ 3. I try to follow the rules.

_____ 4. I go straight for the goal.

_____ 5. I postpone decisions.

_____ 6. I often make last-minute plans.

_____ 7. I excel in what I do.

_____ 8. I like order.

_____ 9. I keep my promises.

_____ 10. I work hard.

_____ 11. I get chores done right away.

_____ 12. I avoid mistakes.

_____ 13. I don't see the consequences of things.

_____ 14. I like to tidy up.

_____ 15. I pay my bills on time.

_____ 16. I turn plans into action.

_____ 17. I have difficulty starting tasks.

_____ 18. I act without thinking.

_____ 19. I handle tasks smoothly.

_____ 20. I want everything to be "just right."

_____ 21. I tell the truth.

_____ 22. I plunge into tasks with all my heart.

_____ 23. I am always prepared.

_____ 24. I choose my words with care.

_____ 25. I have little to contribute.

_____ 26. I love order and regularity.

_____ 27. I listen to my conscience.

_____ 28. I do more than what's expected of me.

_____ 29. I need a push to get started.

_____ 30. I do crazy things.

_____ 31. I don't understand things.

_____ 32. I am not bothered by messy people.

_____ 33. I misrepresent the facts.

_____ 34. I put little time and effort into my work.

_____ 35. I waste my time.

_____ 36. I rush into things.

_____ 37. I am sure of my ground.

_____ 38. I leave my belongings around.

_____ 39. I break rules.

_____ 40. I set high standards for myself and others.

_____ 41. I start tasks right away.

_____ 42. I stick to my chosen path.

_____ 43. I come up with good solutions.

_____ 44. I leave a mess in my room.

_____ 45. I break my promises.

_____ 46. I do just enough work to get by.

_____ 47. I find it difficult to get down to work.

_____ 48. I jump into things without thinking.

_____ 49. I know how to get things done.

_____ 50. I do things according to a plan.

_____ 51. I get others to do my duties.

_____ 52. I demand quality.

_____ 53. I get to work at once.

_____ 54. I make rash decisions.

_____ 55. I misjudge situations.

_____ 56. I often forget to put things back in their proper place.

_____ 57. I do the opposite of what is asked.

_____ 58. I am not highly motivated to succeed.

_____ 59. I carry out my plans.

_____ 60. I like to act on a whim.

Self-efficacy (Se):	1, 7, 13*, 19, 25*, 31*, 37, 43, 49, 55*
Orderliness (Or):	2*, 8, 14, 20, 26, 32*, 38*, 44*, 50, 56*
Dutifulness (Du):	3, 9, 15, 21, 27, 33*, 39*, 45*, 51*, 57*
Achievement-Striving (As):	4, 10, 16, 22, 28, 34*, 40, 46*, 52, 58*
Self-Discipline (Sd):	5*, 11, 17*, 23, 29*, 35*, 41, 47*, 53, 59
Cautiousness (Ca):	6*, 12, 18*, 24, 30*, 36*, 42, 48*, 54*, 60*

NORMS

Se	Or	Du	As	Sd	Ca	TOTAL	PERCENTILE
44	43	48	46	42	39	261	85
40	38	44	42	37	34	233	70
36	32	39	37	31	29	205	50
32	26	34	32	26	24	177	30
28	21	30	28	21	19	145	15

Goldberg, L. R. (1990). An alternative "description of personality": The Big-Five Factor Structure. *Journal of Personality and Social Psychology*. 59, 1216–1229.

1. Based on these assessments, are there links between your personality and your self-assessed professionalism?

2. If you scored low on a personality factor, are there ways you compensate for this weakness? Discuss with your classmates how they deal with their weaknesses.

3. Write a one-page executive summary of the chapter.

4. Review the mind map from the opening of the chapter. Would you change anything after reading the chapter?

What's Important to You in the Chapter?

WITH SEVERAL OF YOUR CLASSMATES, discuss the idea or ideas that are most likely to effect a change in your values, attitudes, or behaviors. Be succinct. Write no more than two sentences. If Blackboard is used in your class, post your important ideas to the site.

References

Kluckhohn, C. M. K., and Murray, H. A. (1953). Personality formation: The determinants. In *Personality in Nature, Culture and Society*. C. M. K. Kluckhorn, H. A. Murray, and D. Schneider, eds. (pp. 53–67). New York: Knopf.

Mayer, J. D. (2007–2008). Personal intelligence. *Imagination, Cognition and Personality*. 27 (3), 209-232.

Nave, C. S., Sherman, R. A., Funder, D. C., Hampson, S. E., and Goldberg, L. R. (2010). On the contextual independence of personality: Teachers' assessments predict directly observed behavior after four decades. *Social Psychology Personality Science*. 3 (1), 1–9.

Tuchman, B. (1981). Is history a guide to the future? In *Practicing History*. New York: Ballantine Books.

Suggested Readings

Borges, N. J., and Gibson, D. D. (2003). Personality patterns of physicians in person-oriented and technique-oriented specialties. *Journal of Vocational Behavior*. 67, 4–20.

Cordina, M., Lauri, M., and Lauri, J. (2010). Patient-oriented personality traits of first-year pharmacy students. *American Journal of Pharmacy Education*. 75 (5, Article 84), 1–7.

Eley, D. S., and Eley, R. M. (2011). Personality traits of Australian nurses and doctors: Challenging stereotypes. *International Journal of Nursing Practice*. 17, 380–387.

Ferguson, E., James, D., and Madeley, L. (2002). Factors associated with success in medical school: Systematic review of the literature. *BMJ*. 324 (April 20), 952–957.

Ferguson, E., Semper, H., Yates, J., Fitzgerald, J. E., Skatova, A., and James, D. (2014). The "dark side" and "bright side" of personality: When too much conscientiousness and too little anxiety are detrimental with respect to the acquisition of medical knowledge and skill. *PLOS One*. 9 (2), 1–11.

Goldberg, L. R. (1990). An alternative "description of personality." The Big Five Structure. *Journal of Personality and Social Psychology*. 59 (6), 1216–1229.

Hall, J., Rosenthal, M., Family, H., Sutton, J., Hall, K., and Tsuyuki, R. T. (2013). Personality traits of hospital pharmacists: Toward a better understanding of factors influencing pharmacy practice change. *Canadian Journal of Hospital Pharmacy*. 66 (5), 289–295.

Holland, J. L. (1997). *Making Vocational Choices: A Theory of Vocational Personalities and Work Environments* (3rd ed). Odessa, FL: Psychological Assessment Resources.

Hunt, K., and Gable, K. N. (2013). Prevalence of depressive symptoms and obsessive-compulsive personality traits among pharmacy students. *Currents in Pharmacy Teaching and Learning*. 5, 541–545.

Lievens, F., Coetsier, P. De Fruyi, F., and De Maeseneer, J. (2002). Medical students' personality characteristics and academic performance: A five-factor model perspective. *Medical Education*. 36, 1050–1056.

Lievens, F., Ones, D., and Dilchert, S. (2009). Personality scale validities increase throughout medical school. *Journal of Applied Psychology*. 94 (6), 1514–1535.

Lifchez, S. D., and Redett, R. J. III. (2014). A standardized patient model to teach and assess professionalism and communication skills: The effect of personality type on performance. *Journal of Surgical Education*. 71 (3, May/June), 297–301.

Mayer, J. D., Panter, A. T., and Caruso, D. R. (2012). Does personal intelligence exist? Evidence from a new ability based measure. *Journal of Personality Assessment*. 94 (2), 124–140.

Mayer, J. D., Wilson, R., and Hazelwood, M. (2010–2011). Personal intelligence expressed: A multiple case study of business leaders. *Imagination, Cognition and Personality*. 30 (2), 201–224.

McManus, I. C., Keeling, A., and Paice, E. (2004). Stress, burnout and doctors' attitudes to work are determined by personality and learning style: A twelve year longitudinal study of UK medical graduates. *BMC Medicine*. 2, 29. www.biomedcentral.com/1741-7015/2/29.

Oda, R., Wataru, M., Shinpei, T., Yuta, K., Mia, T., Toko, K., Yasuyuki, F., and Kai, H. (2014). Personality and altruism in daily life. *Personality and Individual Differences*. 56, 206–209.

Richardson, J. D., Lounsbury, J. W., Bhaskar, T., Gibson, L. W., and Drost, A. W. (2009). Personality traits and career satisfaction of health care professionals. *The Health Care Manager*. 28 (3), 218–226.

Seibert, S. E., and Kraimer, M. L. (2001). The five-factor model of personality and career success. *Journal of Vocational Behavior*. 58, 1–21.

Specht, J., Egloff, B., and Schmukle, S. C. (2011). Stability and change of personality across the life course: The impact of age and major life events on mean-level and rank-order stability of the big five. *Journal of Personality and Social Psychology*. 101 (4), 862–882.

Weinschenk, A. C. (2013). Personality traits and the sense of civic duty. *American Politics Research*. 42 (1), 90–113.

CHAPTER 6

Emotional Intelligence

Preassessment: Emotional Intelligence

Mind Mapping

*Consider the term displayed on the page. For this term, without thinking or editing, write down the ideas, concepts, examples, contradictions, and theories that come to mind. Do not array them in any systematic or orderly manner. Scatter them about the page. Now, draw lines between your additions indicating that there is a relationship between the terms. If something causes something else, indicate this with an arrow. Relationships may be reciprocal, meaning both cause each other, requiring arrows at both ends. Indicate the strength of the relationships by darkening and thickening the lines; stronger relationships have darker and thicker lines. **Most important: There is no right answer. Do not compare with your classmates.** What you have is a mind map, your mental representation of these topics. Review to determine if anything has changed following this section.*

Emotional Intelligence

The Students

I

DANA S. COULDN'T GET THE baby who died on the floor out of her mind or her mother's shriek when Dana told her she was pregnant. She stopped eating for a week, and then she ate four jars of cheese queso dip and chips in one day, moving to a box of chocolates the following day. Dana hated how this made her feel. Normally, Dana exercised three times a week, but she hadn't exercised for three weeks now. Dana noticed how one of her skirts seemed to stretch tighter than normal when she looked at herself in the mirror. She started coming home and going to bed as soon as class was over, usually around 5:00 PM in the afternoon. Dana usually loved everything about Christmas, but this year she just couldn't get into it.

Dana did manage to drag herself out of bed and out to a basketball game and dinner with her boyfriend. He was a great guy. They had been dating since they both arrived on campus the first year. Dana envisioned a future together. Whereas she was shy and reticent, he was outgoing and friendly. He made friends with everyone and was always happy. Everyone liked him. Problems for him seemed to evaporate when he turned on the charm. And if charm didn't work, he just accepted the circumstances as part of life, did the best he could, and moved on. Nothing seemed to bother him.

Right now, though, Dana was so angry with her boyfriend. Although he acknowledged what had happened to her on the floor when the baby died, he told her to get over it. There wasn't anything she could have done. He would listen to her for several minutes as she discussed her feelings, but then he would drift away, either literally or mentally. He told Dana she was acting crazy. This was a sensitive issue with Dana because her mother had suffered a mental breakdown in her early 30s when she lost a baby. Dana broke into tears when her boyfriend got up to talk with one of their female classmates who had come into the restaurant.

II

There he was, the father who had abandoned him, laying in the living room of his apartment, with his mother and sister sitting by his side. Ivan T.'s father had just come back from what was likely to be his final treatment for pancreatic cancer. The end was getting close. They were just waiting to move him to hospice care. He was asleep now. Ivan stood and watched him. Ivan tried to identify all the feelings he had—what they were, whether they were justified, how they had impacted his life, how he couldn't trust anyone, how he tried to make sure he never got hurt in relationships, how he had tried to dull the pain with alcohol, how things were piling up on him at school, how he had never had anyone to turn to for guidance, how he had to work on all his school breaks while his classmates were vacationing, and how cynical and jaded he was at age 23.

Ivan sat down to compose a list of the things he wanted to say to his father. Ivan was fairly certain his father would be relatively lucid for at least a few more days. Ivan wanted to get a few things off of his chest.

III

Before going back to school, Niki M. had eaten in numerous expensive restaurants. She understood good food. She also understood good bar food and good barbecue. In her hometown, one restaurant loaded sandwiches with French fries and coleslaw. It was a long-time tradition. She loved eating there. She appreciated the ambience of a restaurant with white tablecloths as well as one with initials carved in the table. Whatever the ambience, Niki demanded service that was prompt and appropriate. In fact, she expected it. She expected wait staff to go all out; she always did. If she didn't get good service, she would often not a leave a tip, and she would generally chide the wait staff if they did not meet her expectations. Because Niki did not get to go out much anymore, her expectations for good food and service were heightened.

After the last class for the semester, Niki and several of the older students decided to go out to celebrate. One of the other students invited an instructor to attend—the instructor that Niki was attracted to. The choice of restaurants had been difficult; each student had their own preference. The other students outvoted Niki. She knew the choice was not good. She had heard about the restaurant from her parents and knew what to expect. Niki fumed on the drive home. She was right. The food was not good, and the service was poor. During the meal, Niki had been condescending to the wait staff. It was clear from her attitude that she was not happy. Everyone could read it. When the instructor arrived, he had brought a last-minute guest. The instructor's guest had been introduced as a former classmate, but after the dinner, Niki found out she was also a recruiter for a one of the national chains. in the industry. Niki was aware that the chain employed many graduates in her field.

IV

Ryan P. just wanted to watch the hockey game. It was the start of the playoffs. He couldn't remember the last time he indulged himself with this much time not studying. His daughter came and sat down beside him. If he had been more attentive, Ryan would have seen she had something to tell him. Ryan, however, was engrossed in the game. His daughter kept interrupting the game with inane questions and comments. Ryan barely paid attention to her and barely replied to her comments. His responses were perfunctory, the fatherly "Uh huh" to everything. Ryan didn't notice the tears in her eyes until she ran out of the room sobbing. Ryan did not feel any empathy toward her. His only concern was that he knew he would be in trouble with his wife.

⫸ LEARNING OUTCOMES

- Discuss what emotions are.
- Describe emotional intelligence.
- Describe and discuss the four domains of emotional intelligence.
- Discuss emotional hijackings.
- Discuss why emotional intelligence is important.

⫸ KEY TERMS

- Emotions
- Relationship management
- Self-awareness
- Self-management
- Social awareness

What Are Emotions?

EMOTIONS CONTAIN INFORMATION FOR US about what is going on in the world around us. They are tangible. They can be measured in the body. Daniel Goleman, author of the book *Emotional Intelligence* (1995), which brought the idea of emotional intelligence to a larger readership, defines an emotion as "a feeling and its distinctive thoughts, psychological and biological states, and range of propensities to act" (p. 289). Emotions have a cognitive component, a physiological component, and a behavioral component.

What Are the Primary Emotions?

THERE ARE FOUR PRIMARY EMOTIONS recognized around the world, even by preliterate cultures: fear, anger, sadness, and enjoyment. These four emotions, and their variants, can be blended to create innumerable and subtle emotional shadings. Just as artists see shades and hues of color, emotionally astute individuals can understand and describe the shades and hues of their emotional lives. An example of an expanded vocabulary of emotions is detailed below (Data from Goleman 1995).

- **Anger:** Fury, outrage, resentment, wrath, exasperation, indignation, vexation, acrimony, animosity, annoyance, irritability, hostility, and at the extreme, pathological hatred and violence
- **Sadness:** Grief, sorrow, cheerlessness, gloom, melancholy, self-pity, loneliness, dejection, despair, and when pathological, severe depression
- **Fear:** Anxiety, apprehension, nervousness, concern, consternation, misgiving, wariness, qualm, edginess, dread, fright, terror, and as a pathology, phobia and panic
- **Enjoyment:** Happiness, joy, relief, contentment, bliss, delight, amusement, pride, sensual pleasure, thrill, rapture, gratification, satisfaction, euphoria, whimsy, ecstasy, and at the extreme, mania

Simple and Complex Emotions

SOME EMOTIONS ARE SIMPLE AND clean. Fear evoked from seeing a snake in the road is an example. Some emotions are complex and layered. An example of a complex emotional reaction would be a father who, when looking at his newborn baby, is at first ecstatic and then a moment later alarmed and fearful as he realizes there is something wrong with the baby. The circumstance of getting angry because you were angry is another example of a complex and multilayered emotional response. The emotions evoked by either denying or evading our emotions is still another example.

Are Emotions Functional?

EMOTIONS ARE BOTH FUNCTIONAL AND dysfunctional. For example, anger may motivate you to act or alienate you from other people; fear may alert you to a threat or interfere with thinking; sadness may motivate you to reevaluate what you want from life or inhibit you from taking any action at all; and happiness may promote positive relationships or lead you to have unrealistically favorable expectations.

Can I Ignore My Emotions? Can I Hide Them?

EMOTIONS AFFECT EVERYTHING WE DO. We can be mindful of them, we can suppress them, but we cannot ignore them. Emotions work in ways not yet completely understood. Even presumably highly rational decision processes are influenced by our emotional state. Positive and negative moods impact how we decide. Many situations demand that we control or suppress our emotions. The simple fact is that although we can sometimes camouflage our emotions, with more regularity than we suppose, some people read our emotions regularly, and all people read our emotions occasionally.

Why Do I Always React the Same Way?

EACH OF US IS ADDICTED to our emotions. Every morning, we get up and put on our own familiar and comfortable emotional coat. Even though the emotion may be negative and not self-serving, it is the one we choose on a daily basis. This emotional addiction is based on the fact that neurons that fire together create neural networks. These networks reflect the experienced patterns of our emotions, thoughts, and behaviors. This explains why, on a daily basis, a person may tend to feel like a victim, or slightly sad, or optimistic and why similar situations and people always evoke the same emotional response. The neural network is responding as it always does to the same circumstance. Paradoxically, negative emotions like anger and sadness can be strangely comforting due to their familiarity. Although we might be addicted to a specific emotional pattern, we can, with conscious effort, change these patterns.

What Are Moods? What Is Temperament?

EMOTIONS THAT ARE MUTED BUT persist for an extended period (a day or two) are moods, whereas the tendency toward a specific mood over a long time is temperament. For example, you might feel ecstatic for a few moments if someone compliments you, but you might be in a good mood the rest of the day because of the compliment, and if you are naturally happy and content for long periods, that may be your basic disposition or temperament. Emotions arise from identifiable stimuli, whereas moods are feelings that often occur for unknown reasons. Moods may be the "aftershock" of emotional events.

What Is Emotional Intelligence?

EMOTIONAL INTELLIGENCE IS THE ABILITY to understand your emotions and others' emotions and to craft a functional behavior that is suitable to the context. Emotional intelligence does not require that emotions be suppressed or denied; rather, emotions are used to achieve objectives. Some people are better at understanding themselves and the needs of others and building successful and productive relationships. These people are emotionally intelligent.

Is It Really Intelligence or a Skill?

This point is debatable. For our purposes, emotional intelligence is viewed as a skill. From this perspective, levels of emotional intelligence are not fixed but can be increased.

Why Is Emotional Intelligence Important?

As a healthcare worker and someone engaged daily in the complexities of life, death, and practice, understanding and management of one's emotions are essential aspects of personal growth. If certain types of people are emotionally unstable, knowing how to recognize this and defuse it is a professional obligation.

What Are the Domains of Emotional Intelligence?

Emotional intelligence has four domains or core skills: self-awareness, self-management, social awareness, and relationship management. The first two skills, self-awareness and self-management, are primarily about the individual; they are internal. The second two skills, social awareness and relationship management, are about the individual's relationship to the world; they are external.

What Is Self-Awareness?

Self-awareness is the ability to understand who you are. What are your tendencies? What are your emotional reactions to certain circumstances? What type of people upset you? Which challenges energize you? Which intimidate you? What are you afraid of? The potential for self-discovery is unlimited, as experience reveals unfathomed aspects of yourself. The level of self-awareness that is appropriate does not require plumbing the inner depths of your soul and subconscious. Instead, ask yourself in an objective way whether you understand how you operate in the world. Self-awareness is the foundation on which other aspects of emotional intelligence are based.

Why Self-Awareness?

Numerous thinkers have counseled that the formula for development, maturation, and success begins with an accurate picture of one's self and an understanding of how one behaves. In this case, exercises in self-awareness are targeted at personal and professional growth.

What Are the Barriers to Self-Awareness?

There are at least two barriers to acquiring an accurate picture of oneself. One barrier is being faced with information about ourselves that may be too painful or inconsistent with our personal image of who we are. When this information challenges deeply held beliefs about our self and our self-worth, we tend to defend ourselves psychologically by offering explanations and rationales for this discrepancy. The implication of this psychological defense is that it tends to limit our chance for learning and further development.

The second barrier to self-understanding, particularly for healthcare students, is that of time. Self-understanding requires conscious mental energy. It is work. What is gained is only what is put into it. One must take an active role as an observer. The crowded weekly calendar filled with classes, laboratories, study, clinical sites, work, extracurricular activities, and personal relationships simply does not leave the time or the psychic energy for most healthcare students to indulge in the "luxury" of self-observation and self-awareness.

What Is Self-Management?

Self-management is what you do, or do not do, that is appropriate to the context. Context is key. Behaviors appropriate at a student graduation party are ill-advised at a company Christmas party. Self-management requires monitoring your behaviors in specific, discrete circumstances as well as your entrenched tendencies. Self-management requires sublimating your immediate emotional needs for your longer term success. It is difficult to react appropriately in all circumstances; often you will get it wrong. Effective self-management requires self-correction, and the quicker the better.

What Are the Prerequisites for Self-Management?

The first step in self-management is eliminating psychological dissonance in your life. Whenever possible, the things we have to do should be aligned with the things we like to do. If work is a constant irritant and does not meet our inner psychic needs, then we will always be out of sorts. Our emotions will always be close to the surface. Consider how abrupt you might be with someone if you suffered from a toothache all day. Psychic pain caused by a lack of congruence in your life will have the same effect.

The second step in self-management is summed up in this quote by M. Scott Peck, "Life is difficult. This is the great truth, one of the greatest truths—it is a great truth because once we see this truth, we transcend it." Think about your life. Has there ever been a day when you weren't worried about something, afraid of something, or apprehensive about something? To be alive is to have problems and worries. Understanding this, it is easier to keep things in perspective. Although life will have ups and downs, your perspective on these events and your response to those peaks and valleys can smooth out their emotional impact.

What Is at the Core of Self-Management?

The key to self-management is to recognize that you are in control of how you feel and think and how you behave. No other person—let me emphasize, *no one*—makes you feel or think or do anything. Dr. Seuss in *Oh, The Places You'll Go* summed this point as well as anyone. "You have brains in your head. You have feet in your shoes. You can steer yourself any direction you choose. You're on your own and you know what you know. And YOU are the guy who'll decide where to go."

What Is Emotional Regulation and Self-Management?

Emotional regulation is the process by which individuals modulate their emotions. The goal is to control the intensity, duration, occurrence, or expression of emotions. Self-management does not mean that one never feels emotions or lets them show. It would be a cold heart that rounded on a pediatric floor with children suffering from leukemia and felt nothing. Denial of emotions or their universal suppression is not the ideal. A child who violates a mutually agreed upon course of action should see and experience a measure of a parent's displeasure. Feeling emotion is fine, showing emotion is fine, and suppressing emotion is fine. A self-managed individual knows which response is appropriate for any circumstance and can execute the appropriate response. This is a difficult admonition. These situations are subtle, fluid, and multilayered. An expectation that one can be perfect at this is unreasonable. The standard by which to measure oneself on this pursuit is improvement, not perfection.

What Are Specific Strategies for Emotional Regulation?

In managing your emotions and yourself, the following options are available.

- Do not put yourself in situations that you know have the potential to cause you to lose control or focus. Recall what your "hot buttons" are. What are the people, places, and circumstances that over time have caused you to lose your composure? Just stay away from them.
- If you can, alter situations that have the potential of causing you to lose control. If a specific individual gets under your skin, try never to meet with that person alone. The presence of others may moderate your reaction to the person.

- Focus on those aspects of people and circumstances that do not arouse your emotions, rather than the elements that do.
- Reappraise the circumstances that cause emotional turmoil. For example, when taking a critical test, realizing that it is just a series of questions on a piece of paper rather than a measure of your self-worth blunts its emotional power.
- Control and modulate your response to the arousing circumstances. In other words, take a deep breath or walk away for a moment, alter your thought process, and respond rather than react unthinkingly. At the extreme, the emotion is suppressed. If your residency director has a bad day and takes it out on you, it is probably a good idea to quietly take it, rather than lashing back.

The one response that is always in your control is your ability to reappraise circumstances, to frame things in such a way that your emotional response is appropriate.

What Are Emotional Hijackings?

Emotional hijackings, or flashpoints, are circumstances, people, or objects that provoke uncontrolled emotional reactions. Road rage after being cut off in traffic exemplifies an emotional hijacking. Lashing out at someone if you feel belittled is another example. For some, a spider on the wall elicits panic and fear out of proportion to the threat. Emotional hijacking, or reacting without thinking, can be considered a form of emotional *unintelligence*. A significant aspect of emotional intelligence is understanding and managing emotional hijackings.

What Is Social Awareness?

Social awareness requires paying attention to the people and the world around you. You have to look and listen effectively. This requires that you stop talking and stop listening to the internal dialogue in your head. Social intelligence requires seeing people as they are, not as you would like them to be.

What Are Emotions Blinders?

Ironically, although achieving emotional intelligence is the goal, excessive emotions can cloud our judgment, blinding us to social cues in the environment. For example, when you are romantically interested in someone, you often miss the cues the person sends. Although you may be surprised when that person ends the relationship, many of your friends (relatively disinterested and emotionally neutral) will say they could see it coming. Other states of mind also contribute to missing cues when regarding people. One is neediness and is characterized by the saying "Never shop when you are hungry." If you need something more than you would normally or you want something more than another person, then your ability to read people and circumstances is suspect. Fear can also cause you to miss cues. For example, if you are fearful of being alone, you may not notice troubling patterns in the behavior of your significant other. A final state of mind that will inhibit the ability to read people is defensiveness. Once we are engaged in defending our ego against attack or uncomfortable information, we are not likely to notice relevant cues in our environment.

How Can I Improve My Social Awareness?

Social awareness can be improved by using the following techniques:

- **Scan:** At any one time, an overload of information is available for attention and processing. To deal with this issue, first scan the situation. Evaluate the backdrop, the physical aspects of the situation, the room, and the people. In other words, try to see the big picture. After this evaluation, search for subtle clues that might be relevant.
- **Pare:** Next, pare this information down to the aspects that stand out. What catches your eye, your ear, and your other senses? What aspects of this situation pertain directly to the task at hand?
- **Enlarge:** Having identified the specific aspects of the situation most relevant to you, bring these features into sharper focus. Concentrate on these aspects.
- **Evaluate:** Having focused on and determined specific aspects, now evaluate them. Do you see patterns? Are there deviations from normal behaviors? Look for extremes.
- **Decide:** Make a decision based on this process. If possible, test whether your hypothesis is correct. Finally, practice this process as you seek to improve your abilities to read people and situations.

Being socially aware is no different than being an effective clinician. The task is the same; only the context varies. In both cases, the task is to see both the trees and the forest. If a mother calls a pediatrician about a sick child, the pediatrician's questions center on specific markers, such as the child's temperature, whether there is discharge from the nose or a cough, and so on. Ultimately, the doctor will ask the mother whether the child looks sick. In other words, the pediatrician wants specific markers from the mother and a global assessment of the child's condition.

What Is the Critical Element in Reading People?

In the social context, we read vast amounts of information. We explicitly attend to or unconsciously absorb this information. We run mental checklists or intuitively draw conclusions. We analyze the "shows" that people want us to understand about them and their unconscious "tells" that give them away. We process our first and subsequent impressions of people. We will never be completely right in reading someone. What we can do is gather enough information to establish a consistent pattern. If pieces of information about someone present an incongruent picture, then we should be cautious. If our assessment of someone or a situation seems to be congruent or make sense, then this is probably the best we can do.

In developing a consistent, patterned picture of someone's character or emotions, the following points are useful.

- Get a first impression. Form a first impression based on a person's most striking trait. As you acquire more information, confirm or disconfirm your first impressions.
- What is unusual? Extremes and deviations from patterns are important.
- Is the deviation temporary or permanent? People vary on a daily basis; they can be up and down. Is what you are seeing a trend or a single aberrant event?
- Is what you are seeing due to choice or fate? We can all choose to present in many different ways, depending on our needs and circumstances. Nonelective traits have a more pervasive impact on our emotions and behaviors. An extremely small person can choose to dress stylishly and meticulously, but can never escape the shaping influence of stature.

Some traits are more revealing than others. An individual's level of compassion, socioeconomic background, and contentment with life often reveal more about an individual than other traits.

What Is Relationship Management?

We all live in the shadow of one another. Relationships are the key to everything. **Relationship management** builds on the three other emotional intelligence domains. Relationships build over time and take work. Relationships require give and take. Relationship management is a delicate balance between doing things to preserve the relationship and doing things to preserve personal integrity.

Why Is It Hard to Maintain Good Relationships?

Relationships are work. Successful relationships do not just happen. Everyone has a myriad of needs, wants, and aspirations, and some of these may even be subconscious. Inevitably, friction with others sometimes results when people pursue their own needs, wants, and aspirations. A good counsel to keep in mind is that other people are not out to take advantage of you, but they are out for themselves. The key point is that just because a relationship takes work does not mean that it is defective.

If You Are in a Relationship, Shouldn't You Be Selfless?

Regarding the small things, such as what to have for dinner or what color to paint a room, a willingness to accommodate is the lubricant that makes relationships work. However, on core issues, such as how many children to have, attitudes toward money, and career aspirations, the advice is that it is okay to be selfish. Trading away your dreams for a relationship will only beget anger, resentment, and hostility. If individuals are mature, they will work out their differences; if not, then the resentments will emerge surreptitiously. Ultimately, core issues will need to be addressed or the relationship will end or become a hollow shell populated by two cynical and disinterested parties.

If They Would Only…

A familiar refrain in dealing with another person is something like, "Things would be okay if you would just… ." Implicit in this comment is the notion that the relationship would improve if the other person would change. And if they will not change, your task is to change them to suit your needs. This misses the key point regarding change in humans: you can never change another person. If the relationship is difficult and in trouble, the only aspect that you control is yourself. If you change, then the other person will change. Reciprocity accounts for this phenomenon. If you want someone to be more considerate of your feelings, then be considerate of theirs. If you want someone to be more open about their issues, then be open about your issues. You are only responsible for you; you are not responsible for the other person's behavior.

What Is Reciprocity?

The essence of any relationship is two people trying to get what they want. Successful relationships are based on a psychological contract of supportive reciprocity. In other words, you will get from someone whatever you give to someone.

What Are My Rights in the Relationship?

To maintain and strengthen relationships, we must assert ourselves in an appropriate manner. Passive acceptance and disregard is not the path to a functioning relationship. In asserting ourselves, regarding the relationship, it is permissible to ask for what you want, it is okay to say no, and you must negotiate conflict without damaging the relationship. In strengthening and maintaining relationships, it is helpful to understand the "rights" that both of you have in the relationship. Those rights are to need things, to be first sometimes, to ask for help, to say no, and to sometimes inconvenience or disappoint.

What Is Transference?

A key point regarding relationships is the understanding that no relationship is new. All current relationships are colored by previous relationships. The term for this phenomenon is transference, and it occurs at an unconscious level. Humans' most potent relationships are with their earliest caregivers. These early relationships are internalized and idealized. The first "organization" for all of us is the family. It is the notion of transference that explains why if, for example, a woman had an autocratic father who was overbearing, she now finds herself inexplicably arguing with her male boss. She unconsciously acts as if her boss was her father. If you have ever taken an instant dislike to someone for no apparent reason other than the way he or she looks and acts, then transference is the likely explanation.

What Is a Toxic Relationship?

Sometimes people find themselves in a toxic relationship, one where they are asked to sacrifice all of their needs for the enrichment of the other. Such relationships are best exemplified by cult leaders. In personal relationships, extreme infatuation with another person leads an individual to sacrifice everything to maintain the relationship. There is a sense of complete fulfillment. No other human can completely fulfill your needs. Insecurity and the need to feel special drive such a relationship. Needless to say, toxic relationships do not turn out well for at least one of the parties. Toxic relationships are best avoided.

What Characterizes a Successful Relationship?

Long-term successful relationships are characterized by the following (Data from Tamm and Luyet 2004, p. 9):

- **Collaborative intent.** Partners to a relationship make a mutual commitment to the relationship.
- **Truthfulness.** Partners commit to both telling and listening to the truth. This is accomplished by creating an atmosphere of openness and trust where the difficult issues can be considered.
- **Self-accountability.** Partners accept responsibility for their lives, the choices they make, and the consequences of their choices. Accountability trumps blaming.
- **Awareness of self and others.** Partners to the relationship commit to enhancing self-awareness and understanding the context of their circumstances and issues that motivate others.
- **Problem solving.** Partners to the relationship commit to engaging in effective problem solving rather than subtle competition.

Successful relationships are collaborations between people in pursuit of mutually beneficial goals.

Conclusion

THIS CHAPTER INTRODUCED THE IDEA of emotional intelligence, which is the ability to understand your emotions and the emotions of others and then craft a behavior appropriate to the context. It discusses the four domains of emotional intelligence: self-awareness, self-management, social awareness, and relationship management.

What Do the Practitioners/Others Say?

FOR NEXT CLASS, BE PREPARED to discuss emotions and emotional intelligence based on any *one* of the following:

- A discussion with your colleagues, or others, on how they feel and what they know about emotional intelligence.
- An article on emotional intelligence, either from the research literature or any other source.
- A movie, television program, or YouTube video about emotional intelligence.
- A book on emotional intelligence (literary, historical, psychological, or any other source).

Personal Learning Plan: Emotional Intelligence

USE THE FOLLOWING GUIDE TO develop a personal and professional growth project.

What prompted you to develop this plan?	
What is the general area for improvement?	
What is the specific issue for improvement?	
Why is this important to you?	
How do you generally act in these areas?	
What are your goals?	
What strategies are required?	
Who/what is necessary to meet your goals with this strategy?	
How will you measure success/failure with this effort?	
How will you reflect and capture the lesson from this effort that can be generalized to other circumstances?	

The Students: Personal and Professional Issues

B ASED ON THE DESCRIPTION OF each student at the beginning of the chapter, what are the personal and professional issues (either immediately or in the future) confronting each student? Consider whether they are linked and, if so, how. Finally, what would you recommend to each student to resolve these issues?

Dana S.

Personal Issues

Professional Issues

Are They Linked? Will the Personal Issues Impact Professional Behavior?

Recommendations

Ivan T.

Personal Issues

Professional Issues

Are They Linked? Will the Personal Issues Impact Professional Behavior?

Recommendations

Niki M.

Personal Issues

Professional Issues

Are They Linked? Will the Personal Issues Impact Professional Behavior?

Recommendations

Ryan P.

Personal Issues

Professional Issues

Are They Linked? Will the Personal Issues Impact Professional Behavior?

Recommendations

Exercises

Who Are My Emotional Role Models?

Our attitudes toward our emotions are derived from our experiences with our earliest caregivers, typically family. Those we meet during childhood and adolescence shape our emotional world. Take a few moments to identify your emotional role models by answering the following questions.

1. What positive emotional traits did you pick up from your mother and/or father?

2. What negative emotional trait did you pick up from your mother and/or father?

What Are My Emotional Triggers?

All of us have people and situations that provoke strong emotional reactions. Take a moment to consider what your emotional triggers are.

1. Describe a time when you lost control of your emotions. What was the precipitating event?

2. Is there a pattern to when you lose control of your emotions?

3. What triggers cause you to lose your composure?

Describe Your Emotions

1. What does it feel like to be in love?

2. What does it feel like when you break up with someone?

3. What does it feel like when someone breaks up with you?

Emotional Catalog

For the next week, keep a record of your emotions, the events that caused them, their length, and their impact on the day.

Date	Emotion	Circumstances (What happened? What was going on that day?)
Monday		
Tuesday		
Wednesday		
Thursday		
Friday		
Saturday		
Sunday		

Based on this log, do you see any patterns? Are these patterns helpful or not?

How Would You Rate Your Emotional Intelligence?

Ask yourself the following questions, assigning a rating from poor to good. If possible, also ask someone close to you to answer the questions on your behalf. That external perspective will help prevent self-reporting bias. Rate yourself from 1 to 10 on these points, with 1 being poor and 10 being good.

1. How good are you at understanding others from their perspective? _____

2. How sensitive are you about the feelings of others? _____

3. Do you easily make friends? _____

4. Are you willing to express your emotions to others? _____

5. Are you good at solving conflicts? _____

6. Can you easily adapt your behavior to changing circumstances? _____

7. Does your behavior invite other people's expression of warmth toward you? _____

8. Do you perceive the impact you have on others (even if no reaction is expressed)? _____

9. When you are confronted with a perplexing situation, are you able to handle it? _____

10. Can you easily deal with people who ask you questions about your personal life? _____

11. Are you good at seeking out others to help you when the need arises? _____

12. Do you routinely reflect on your actions? _____

If you (and others) consistently rate you on the high end of the scale, you are lucky—it sounds as if you have a high EQ, or emotional intelligence. If not, you should put some effort into the further development of this crucial part of human functioning.

Kets de Vries, M. (2001). *The Leadership Mystique*. London: Pearson Education Limited.

Emotional Type

All of us have a particular style of relating to our emotions and to the world. This is the filter through which we see the world. Understanding our type helps us understand how we behave in the world. Our emotional type is due to inborn temperament and parental influence. No single type is superior to another. Understanding your emotional type is a key element to developing your emotional intelligence. It is a key aspect of self-awareness, but only a beginning. Emotional type can evolve over time. Also, most of us are combinations of several emotional types. See if any of the types below are a match for you.

The Intellectual

Intellectuals live in their head. They are cerebral. The world is seen through a rational filter. Intellectuals are at risk of being cut off from their emotions.

The Empath

Empaths feel everything. They have a finely tuned antenna for emotions. For the empath, intuition is the filter for their world.

The Rock

Rocks are emotionally strong. They are practical. They are cool. They care about your pain but maintain their boundaries. They like life on an even keel but will deal with life's problems. Rocks internalize their emotions.

The Gusher

Gushers are the opposite of rocks, they are intimately in tune with their emotions and want to share them. They tend to be spontaneous and authentic. Gushers unload stress by verbalizing it.

Data from Orloff, J. (2009). *Emotional Freedom*. New York: Harmony Books.

Perspective

1. Describe the biggest emotional crisis of your high school years. How important is this event to you now?

2. Describe the biggest emotional event of your college career. How important is it to you now?

3. Write down your grade point average and class standing. How important do you think it will be in 20 years?

4. If you were given a terminal diagnosis today, what event in your past life would still be important today?

Examine Your Beliefs

With several classmates, discuss and isolate the collective belief about performance on a test. Also with several classmates, discuss and isolate the collective belief about talking in class. Do these beliefs meet the test for effective thinking? Specifically, do they meet an empirical test (Is there proof that these beliefs are true?), a functional test (Do these beliefs help you or make things worse?), or a logical test (Do they meet a test for common sense?)?

Who Is a Millionaire?

As an exercise in social awareness, go to any location and try and pick out who is the millionaire or who has the most money.

What's Really Going On?

Watch a movie with the sound off and try to determine what is happening in the scene.

Who Is Romantically Interested?

How do you tell if someone is romantically interested in you?

Am I Active or Passive in Relationships?

Do you try and get along no matter what, or do you take charge of the relationship?

Your Relationship Foundations

1. How did your parents model relationships for you?

2. How did your family respond to you when you communicated an emotional need?

3. Were you encouraged to express your needs while growing up? If so, how?

4. As a child, how did you get others to respond to your needs?

5. As an adult, how do you get others to respond to your needs?

6. Do your emotions get in the way of expressing your needs? How do you handle it when someone does not honor your request to have a need met?

Data from Spradling, S. E. (2003). *Don't Let Your Emotions Run Your Life* (pp. 144–146). Oakland, CA: New Harbinger Publications.

Summarize

1. Write a one-page executive summary of the chapter.

2. Review the mind map from the opening of the chapter. Would you change anything following reading the chapter?

What's Important to You in the Chapter?

WITH SEVERAL OF YOUR CLASSMATES, discuss the idea or ideas most likely to effect a change in your values, attitudes, or behaviors. Be succinct. Write no more than two sentences.

References

Goleman, D. (1995). *Emotional Intelligence.* New York: Bantam Dell.

Tamm, J. W., and Luyet, R. J. (2004). *Radical Collaboration.* New York: Collins Business.

Suggested Readings

Ablom, M. (19970). *Tuesdays with Morrie.* New York: Random House.

Beitman, B., Viamontes, G., Soth, A., and Nittler, J. (2006). Toward a neural circuitry of engagement, self-awareness, and pattern search. *Psychiatric Annals.* 36 (4), 272–282.

Brach, T. (2003). *Radical Acceptance*. New York: Bantam Books.

Bradberry, T., and Greaves, J. (2009). *Emotional Intelligence 2.0.* San Diego, CA: Talent Smart.

Bricker, D., Young, J. E., and Flanagan, C. M. (1993). Schema-focused cognitive therapy: A comprehensive framework for characterological problems. In *Cognitive Therapies in Action*. K. T. Kuehlwein and H. Rosen, eds. San Francisco, CA: Jossey-Bass.

Caruso, D. R., and Salovey, P. (2004). *The Emotionally Intelligent Manager.* San Francisco, CA: Jossey-Bass.

Dimitrius, J. E., and Mazzarella, W. P. (2008). *Reading People*. New York: Ballantine Books.

Epstein, S. (1998). *Constructive Thinking: The Key to Emotional Intelligence.* West Port, CT: Praeger.

Friday, P. J. (1999). *Friday's Laws*. Pittsburgh, PA: Bradley Oak Publications.

Gardner, H. (2004). *Frames of Mind: The Theory of Multiple Intelligences.* New York: Basic Books.

Glasser, W. (1985). *Positive Addiction*. New York: Harper and Rowe.

Gross, J. J., and Thompson, R. A. (2007). Emotion regulation. In *Handbook of Emotion Regulation*. James J. Gross, ed. New York: The Guilford Press.

Hayashi, A. M. (2001). When to trust your gut. *Harvard Business Review.* February, 59–65.

Hodgkinson, G. P., Langan-Fow, J., and Sadler-Smith, E. (2008). Intuition: A fundamental bridging construct in the behavioral sciences. *British Journal of Psychology.* 99, 1–27.

Kasar, J., and Clark, E. N. (2000). *Developing Professional Behaviors*. Thorofare, NJ: Slack Inc.

Kets de Vries, M. (2001). *The Leadership Mystique*. London: Pearson Education Limited.

Mayer, J. D., Salovey, P., and Caruso, D. R. (2004). A further consideration of the issues of emotional intelligence. *Psychological Inquiry* 15 (3), 249–255.

McKay, M., Wood, J. C., and Brantley, J. (2007). *The Dialectical Behavior Therapy Skills Workbook*. Oakland, CA: New Harbinger Publications.

McKenna, J. A. (2005). *Beyond Tells: Power Poker Psychology*. New York: Kensington Publishing.

Orloff, J. (2009). *Emotional Freedom*. New York: Harmony Books.

Peck, M. S. (2003). *The Road Less Traveled*. New York: Simon and Schuster.

Segal, J. (1997). *Raising Your Emotional Intelligence: A Practical Guide*. New York: Owl Books.

Schutte, N. S., Manes, R. R., and Malouff, J. M. (2009). Antecedent-focused emotion regulation, response modulation and well-being. *Current Psychology.* 28, 21–31.

Spradlin, S. E. (2003). *Don't Let Your Emotions Run Your Life.* Oakland, CA: New Harbinger Publications.

Szasz, P. L., Szentagotai, A., and Hofmann, S. G. (2001). The effect of emotion regulation strategies on anger. *Behavior Research and Therapy.* 49, 114–119.

CHAPTER 7

Thinking and Cognition

Andrea Pfalzgraf, PhD, Co-author

Preassessment: Thinking and Cognition

Mind Mapping

Consider the term displayed on the page. For this term, without thinking or editing, write down the ideas, concepts, examples, contradictions, and theories that come to mind. Do not array them in any systematic or orderly manner. Scatter them about the page. Now, draw lines between your additions, indicating that there is a relationship between the terms. If something causes something else, indicate this with an arrow. Relationships may be reciprocal, meaning both cause each other, requiring arrows at both ends. Indicate the strength of the relationships by darkening and thickening the lines; stronger relationships have darker and thicker lines. **Most important: There is no right answer. Do not compare with your classmates.** *What you have is a mind map, your mental representation of these topics. Review to determine if anything has changed following this section.*

Wisdom

The Students

I

DANA S. FINALLY HAD TO acknowledge that her reluctance to speak up and her shyness were a problem. She was always so afraid of offending someone. Her refrigerator was always full of leftovers from restaurant dinners because she thought she would offend the server if she didn't eat all of her food or at least take it home. Dana couldn't count the number of leftover meals she had thrown out or the number of meals she had paid for that were just awful. Any reasonable person would have asked for a refund.

Two things had happened at work recently. Whenever anyone asked to switch schedules, Dana always accommodated the request, regardless of the imposition to her. Generally, people would reciprocate the favor if she asked them. One colleague had asked to switch the schedule four times in the last month. Dana liked to help her colleague because she was planning her wedding. Twice Dana had asked for the favor in return and been denied. One time she had to miss a concert that she had tickets for. Dana saw an email from the offending colleague asking for another switch. It seemed that the colleague assumed Dana would make the switch. She didn't ask Dana if she had any plans and even made allusions to Dana's lack of a social life.

Dana prided herself on her concern for her patients and her attentiveness to their needs and to those of their families. If asked, Dana would do almost anything to improve their experience. The daughter of an elderly patient had just gone too far. She yelled at Dana, told her she was just hired help, demeaned her professional qualifications, and even though Dana solved the situation, continued the rant for 2 hours. The last time Dana had seen the daughter, she started yelling again. Legitimate complaints were one thing, but abuse was quite another.

Dana heard her mother's refrain, "One is always a lady; be gracious."

II

Ivan T. had always lived by one simple rule: never trust anyone. A corollary to that rule was to never let anyone see you hurt or vulnerable. Whenever Ivan met someone, he was aloof and appraising. He checked them out to determine what their angle was or how they might take advantage of him.

He never hugged anyone. In fact, when his 4-year-old nephew tried to hug him, he turned him away saying, "I never hug." All of his personal relationships had ended with the other person leaving, claiming he was cold, aloof, and afraid of intimacy. When he met someone new, he never talked about his life or his father, only declaring that he had a less than ideal childhood. Each breakup confirmed his rule; never trust anyone.

It was a great rule, but Ivan was lonely. His only friends, acquaintances really, were the people at the gym. Ivan knew he was described as aloof and arrogant. He was perceptive enough to understand that this would be a handicap in his career. He had ample evidence that it was a problem in his personal life. Recently, Ivan began to watch how the people at the gym interacted. Although all were focused, two caught his attention by taking time to chat with the other members. Everyone seemed to be glad to see them. One was a woman, about Ivan's age, who appeared to be suffering from some type of neurological disease. She had a slight tremor in her legs. Ivan marveled at how she would just ask total strangers if she could work out with them and how easily she could make everyone laugh. Didn't she know how vulnerable she was?

III

Niki M. had upped the miles she was running each week. The good news was that she was losing weight and her clothes fit better. For some reason, the extra mileage had caused her feet to change. Her customary shoe size, the one she had worn since adolescence, was now too small. Her legs were starting to cramp because her shoes were too tight, so she went to buy herself a new pair of running shoes.

Over the last 3 weeks, Niki had been having a problem with her son. Niki knew he was spoiled. She felt guilty about the time she spent away from him, both while she was in school and now while she was getting her career started. Plus, her new relationship was taking time away from her son. Like most parents who feel guilty, Niki tried to assuage the guilt by buying her son things. Generally, he was appreciative. But now, he was demanding and expected to be bought things whenever they were out. They had clashed for the last 3 weeks. She had sent him to his room several times. Quite frankly, Niki found his demands burdensome. Didn't he know she needed some time for herself?

Standing in line to pay for her running shoes, Niki noticed an attractive young mother with a boy in a wheelchair who was about 4 years older than her son. The boy was severely handicapped. He appeared to be blind, was on oxygen, and had serious skeletomuscular deformities. He was dressed in the latest fashion.

As the mother pushed him out of the store, she stopped and whispered in his ear and blew on his lips. The boy smiled. Niki went to her car and cried, ashamed of what she had been thinking.

IV

Ryan P. had been raised to take care of things, to fix things. His father was like that, and he admired him for it, even though he wasn't very good at it. His father tried, and he cared. Ryan tried to model that behavior. Lately, he had clashed with everyone is his life. His two daughters were barely speaking to him, and when they did, the conversation was laced with sarcasm. Since Ryan lost his job and his income, his wife had gone back to work full time. Now her income exceeded his. Ryan and his mother were fighting over the next step in the care for his father, who was in the early stages of Alzheimer disease.

The latest incident occurred at school during a group project. Another student, who, like Ryan, was an older working adult, was hijacking their group project. She had also been a corporate executive and was running the sessions and treating Ryan and the other students in the group like her staff. Without consulting anyone, she had written the project for the entire group and asked for everyone to comment and then sign off on the project for submission. Ryan admitted that it was a good effort, but he was bothered that he had not made a significant contribution and he didn't like not being in control. The choice now was whether to approve the work or not. The other group members didn't want his advice.

⚜ LEARNING OBJECTIVES

- Discuss expertise and how it relates to personal and professional growth.
- Describe intuition, judgment, wisdom, practical thinking, and stupidity.
- Describe the Six Hat Thinking Method.
- Discuss whether thinking is rational.

✤ KEY TERMS

- Analytical thinking
- Expertise
- Intuition
- Judgment
- Practical intelligence
- Stupidity
- Wisdom

"The goal of effective living is to think effectively: to know when we have crazy ideas."

Friday 1999, Preface, p 15

Mind Mapping

EACH CHAPTER BEGINS WITH AN exercise in mind mapping as a preassessment. These maps represent the internal schema or mental models for the topic under discussion. The maps capture the beliefs of an individual about a topic and the individual's understanding of how, and to what degree, the beliefs are related. In essence, they are a visual representation of what an individual thinks about a certain topic. Mind maps make explicit (to the extent possible) the hidden nuances of an individual's beliefs of their thinking. Mind maps represent current thinking; with experience, a practitioner who takes the time to reflect on his or her performance should develop richer and more nuanced mind maps. In other words, mind maps can be integral aids to continued professional and personal growth.

Thinking

WE ALL KNOW WHAT THINKING is. It is what goes on inside our head when we try to solve problems. Cognitive psychology seeks to understand the way people think, the way they remember things, the way they judge, the way they know, and the way they problem solve. People who think better are deemed to be more intelligent. Intelligence is one's capacity for logic, abstract thought, understanding, self-awareness, communication, learning, emotional knowledge, memory, planning, creativity, and problem solving. Intelligence is general mental capability involving the ability to reason, plan, solve problems, think abstractly, comprehend complex ideas, learn quickly, and learn from experience. Intelligence involves more than the linguistic and mathematical skills of typical intelligence tests. It reflects a broader and deeper capability for comprehending our surroundings—"catching on," "making sense" of things, or "figuring out" what to do.

Learning how one thinks is an avenue for personal and professional growth. Individuals need to understand whether they panic under pressure (stop thinking) or choke (overthink). Do they think up excuses if they make a mistake? Do they think of their patients as insurance claims or human beings? Can they think through a problem if they do not have a clear-cut protocol available? Do they think being professional is more important than making money? Do they think they have arrived educationally or that graduation signals a completion? Do they think they can or cannot change? Do they think the other professionals they interact with are smarter or more qualified? Everything a professional does involves thinking.

There are many types of thinking: clinical, rational, faulty, delusional, systems, realistic, creative, strategic, linear, abstract, theoretical, disciplined, and magical. There are as many types of thinking as there are problems to be solved. Healthcare practice obviously involves clinical thinking as a core. Two predominant assumptions of clinical thinking are that it should be based on evidence and that the decision process should be rational and scientific. Both perspectives are useful, doing much to elevate practice. The fact is, however, that they neglect certain aspects of how people actually think. The human brain did not evolve as an organ to calculate probabilities or make statistical inferences. The human brain evolved as an organ for survival. Human thinking and decision making are subject to well-known biases and traps. Examples of these include the following (Data from Hammond, Keeney, and Raiffa 2006):

- **The anchoring trap.** The human mind inordinately focuses on the first impressions, information, and data that it receives. Subsequent decisions are then anchored to this initial impression. Anchors include comments by a colleague, a statistic in an article, stereotypes about people, and historical trends or events. If the first clinical recommendation you make results in an idiosyncratic reaction, in subsequent recommendations, you will always factor in this consequence, whether appropriate or not.

- **The status quo trap.** Humans display a strong bias for things as they are. To make a change incurs personal responsibility and the possibility of criticism and derision. Following an accepted protocol protects the clinician from rebuke and liability. The problem is that protocols become outdated, may not apply to this patient, or may be only marginally effective.

- **The sunk cost trap.** The sunk cost trap involves continuing to pursue a course of action that you recommended even though that course of action is not working. It is the idea of throwing good money after bad. The sunk cost trap is persistence taken to an illogical and ineffective conclusion.

- **The confirming evidence trap.** In making decisions, humans have a tendency to look for information that confirms their point of view or predetermined choice. Information that does not support our point of view is discounted.

- **The framing trap.** How a decision choice is framed significantly impacts the choices made. Choices framed as a gain rather than a loss will impact the decision. Saying a drug has a 90% success rate begets one decision. Saying it has a 1 in 1,000 chance of causing a fatal brain infection may beget a different decision.

- **The overconfidence trap.** Most of us overrate our abilities; we all tend to believe we are above average.

- **The prudence trap.** In the prudence trap, we adjust our best estimate to include a "fudge" factor just to be safe. If we believe a 10-day course of treatment is correct, we will recommend 12 days just to be certain.

- **The recallability trap.** Anything that distorts or enhances your ability to recall information in a balanced way will bias future choices. A fatal error with a patient will never be forgotten and will likely impact our clinical decisions for a lifetime.

There are numerous other biases in human thinking, far beyond what is required for this chapter. This brief list is just to introduce the idea that, as a professional, your decision-making process may be less than optimal because, like all humans, your thinking is flawed. This is true in the clinical arena as well as for personal and professional growth. Consider the status quo trap. The recognition that people tend toward inertia, to maintain what they already know, is a powerful insight into understanding personal growth, or lack thereof. The only defense against these biases is to be aware of them and to test and retest your choices with rigor and discipline.

Analytical Thinking

ANALYTICAL THINKING IS DELIBERATE AND conscious. We know we are doing it and can describe how we do it. Working through a case in order to make a recommendation based on the observable, concrete physical and clinical evidence is an example of analytical thinking. It is the process of being scientific and rational. A case analysis methodology is detailed next.

Case Analysis: A Tool to Help You Think

A TIME-HONORED WAY TO THINK THROUGH a problem is the case analysis approach. The mechanics of this process are as follows:

Step 1: Identify the problem.

Step 2: Assess by collecting history and physical data.

Step 3: Formulate competing hypotheses, diagnoses, alternatives, and so on.

Step 4: Gather additional information and conduct research in support of each hypothesis, diagnosis, or alternative.

Step 5: Select a specific hypothesis, diagnosis, or alternative as correct.

Step 6: Develop a plan of action.

Step 7: Implement and evaluate the choice.

Here are some tips on case analysis (Data from De Bono 1994).

1. Read through the case quickly to get a general impression of the problem. Highlight any points that jump out. Begin to formulate the problem.

2. To focus attention, use the following devices.

   a. Consider All Factors (CAF): Ask yourself whether all the important factors have been considered.

   b. Other People's Views (OPV): How would another clinician look at this same problem? Is there an alternative view of the problem?

    c. Plus, Minus, Interesting (PMI): Which facts support your hypothesis, which facts do not, and which facts are interesting but irrelevant?

3. In making the decision, use the following aids.

    a. Clarify what the purpose of the decision is; in working through the choices, remain focused on this purpose.

    b. What are the short-term and long-term consequences of the choices?

    c. If the problem is approached from another person's point of view, what would the decision be?

    d. Is it possible to look at the problem from a different perspective?

    e. Does the proposed choice violate or support your values?

What Is Intuition?

IN CONTRAST TO ANALYTICAL THINKING, thinking that is unconscious and rapid is intuitive. We cannot describe how we do this type of thinking; it just happens. Recommendations that begin with, "I have a feeling" are examples of intuitive thinking. **Intuition** is the "affectively charged judgments that arise through rapid, nonconscious, and holistic associations" (Dane and Platt 2009, p. 4). In contrast, the conscious processing of problems is deliberate, rational, and sequential. Intuition has a role in how problems are solved, as input to moral decisions, and as an aid in creativity where multiple elements are fused in a creative synthesis. Intuition is often described as a gut feeling, instinct, common sense, or a premonition. Much high-level thinking is intuitive, operating like the autopilot in a jet liner without conscious involvement or attention. The fictional character Sherlock Holmes described how he solved a problem as follows: "From long habit the train of thoughts ran so swiftly through my mind that I arrived at the conclusion without consciousness of the intermediate steps" (Greenhalg 2002, p. 396). Intuition involves pattern recognition, similarity recognition, common sense understanding, and a sense of salience. In a clinical context, involvement with the patient and the patient's care aids in intuition.

Is Intuition Inferior or Superior to Other Modes of Thinking?

INTUITION IS NEITHER INFERIOR NOR superior to other modes of thinking. It is, however, likely to be more effective in certain instances. Those circumstances are when the decision maker is more experienced and confident; when tasks involve judgments with no objective criteria but have political, ethical, aesthetic, or behavioral overtones; and when time is short.

What Is Judgment?

JUDGMENT IS THE ABILITY TO "infer, estimate, and predict the character of unknown events" (Hastie and Dawes 2001, p. 48). Judgment is the thinking process used when you do not have all the information. Imagine trying to predict the true biological age of a patient only from the visibly apparent cues. Characteristics such as hair color, body movement, skin tone and texture, clothes, and voice are all cues that are used to make this judgment. From these cues, the age of the patient is estimated. In a clinical context, a significant literature may exist on a disease state along with a significant literature on a drug. As long as the patient fits the accepted profile on which this information is based, a clinical decision is straightforward. However, if a particular patient is outside this known profile (e.g., is morbidly obese or has an unusual comorbidity), then a therapeutic choice and outcome can only be inferred or estimated. Beginning a recommendation with a phrase such as "My best guess" is an indicator of judgment.

What Is Practical Intelligence?

PRACTICAL INTELLIGENCE IS THE PRAGMATIC know-how to get things done. The ideal protocol is one thing, whereas the practical protocol, one that is actually feasible, is another; one is a theory, the other is a plan. The knowledge of how to get things done is based on the acquisition of the complex rules of how the organization and people work in a specific context. Generally, these rules are not openly expressed or explicitly taught. It is up to the individual to read the subtle cues and make the appropriate inferences. Learning in this fashion is termed tacit learning and is the foundation of practical intelligence. The ease with which one acquires this practical knowledge is a measure of one's practical intelligence. A clinician lacking in the practical knowledge to get things done cannot be considered an expert. The practical knowledge of how drugs flow through the system, which departments and personalities facilitate or impede this flow, how the drugs get paid for, and how adherent the patient is likely to be is embedded and inseparable from any medication therapy program. For the pharmacist, practical intelligence regarding the distribution function and mastery of that process is inherent in the journey to expertise.

What Is Stupidity?

STUPIDITY IS THE RESULT OF not thinking. It is not a measure of intelligence or capability, because truly smart people often do stupid things. Stupidity is a result of thinking becoming frozen. Excessive adherence to rules, protocols, and internal schema in the face of evidence is stupidity. Stupidity is the "learned corruption of learning" (Welles 1991, p. 1). Stupidity is the " unquestioning acceptance of any one set of constraints or axioms that algorithmically 'determine' the problem-solving steps one needs to take in order to produce the desired behavior" (Moldoveanu and Langer 2002, p. 229). An effective technique for dealing with stupidity is to ask yourself: why are we doing it this way? If the answer is because we have always done it this way, rather than because it produces the best results, then caution is in order. In the movie *Duck Soup*, Chico Marx captured this idea when he said, "Who are you going to believe, me or your own eyes?" It is the objective evidence that determines whether a decision is correct. It is not the unwavering adherence to protocol.

What Is Wisdom?

WISDOM HAS BEEN AN ELUSIVE concept of interest to humans since antiquity. Wisdom may be defined as "the application of tacit knowledge as mediated by values toward the goal of achieving a common good (a) through a balance among multiple intrapersonal, interpersonal, and extrapersonal interests" (Sternberg 1998). The key aspect of this definition is the idea of balancing competing interests. An alternative definition of wisdom is "expertise in the fundamental pragmatics of life" (Baltes and Staudinger 2000, p. 124). This definition rests on the idea of an understanding of the essence of the human condition and the conduct of a good life. The following criteria outline the nature of wisdom (Data from Baltes and Staudinger 2000):

- Wisdom addresses important and difficult questions and strategies about the conduct and the meaning of life.
- Wisdom includes knowledge about the limits of knowledge and the uncertainties of the world.
- Wisdom represents a truly superior level of knowledge, judgment, and advice.
- Wisdom constitutes knowledge with extraordinary scope, depth, measure, and balance.
- Wisdom involves a perfect synergy of mind and character, that is, an orchestration of knowledge and virtues.
- Wisdom represents knowledge used for the good or well-being of oneself and that of others.
- Wisdom is easily recognized when manifested, although difficult to achieve and to specify.

Those who are wise have a rich factual knowledge about life; a rich procedural knowledge about life; an understanding of the issues related to each stage of life; an understanding of life's priorities and what is valuable; and an understanding that life is uncertain. Wisdom is the art of living—of living a life that is beneficial to oneself, others, and society at large. Wisdom is an understanding of what is important.

What Is Expertise? Who Is an Expert?

A PROFESSIONAL SCHOOL IS A DELIBERATE attempt to create an expert. **Expertise** can be shown in skills, knowledge, or abilities or in processes such as personal and professional growth. An expert is someone who demonstrates expertise. Cognitively, experts possess extensive and up-to-date content knowledge, highly developed perceptual abilities, a sense of what is relevant, an ability to simplify complex problems, an ability to adapt to exceptions, and an ability to perceive meaningful patterns in large masses of information; they are faster, have superior long-term and short-term memories, see problems at a deeper level, can anticipate, have a global view of the situation, and have a richer repertoire of strategies. In other words, someone expert in personal and professional growth can take the complexities of life and practice, extract the appropriate lessons, think about those lessons effectively, and then use those lessons to elevate their life and practice.

Experts get to places faster with less effort. The reason for this is that experts have a pretested, preloaded script, or mental blueprint, of how to get there. As a result, experts do not have to stop and consciously work through the process step by step or consciously recall or consult basic principles that underlie the process. Experience provides experts with knowledge of what something is or how something works; they do not need to consciously remember the details of how this knowledge was obtained. For example, imagine driving in a major city you have never been to before and having to locate a destination. Even with a map or a GPS system, you will likely look for and double-check the street signs and drive cautiously to avoid missing a turn. You may even slow down to admire the architecture and ruminate on the nuances of how the city is laid out. You will get to your destination eventually. However, problems arise if traffic patterns are disrupted due to construction that is not reflected on the map or in the GPS system. In contrast, someone who drives in this city everyday will likely be on autopilot, knowing where the bottlenecks are and paying attention to only a few critical turns and merges. Having driven in the city daily, the city's architecture no longer attracts the driver unless it is significantly altered. Even unanticipated bottlenecks are easily negotiated as several alternative routes are known. The experienced driver gets there as quickly and as easily as possible.

What Are the Stages of Expertise?

THE VIEW TAKEN HERE IS that expertise is a developmental process. People are not born experts; they develop into experts. Again, our purpose is in developing greater expertise in personal and professional growth, particularly as it relates to an individual's thinking. The development of expertise goes through stages. The Model of Domain Learning (MDL) posits three stages in expertise development. Acclimation is the initial stage. In this stage, learners orient (acclimate) themselves to a complex and unfamiliar domain. The learner has limited and fragmented knowledge of the domain. The next stage is competence, where the learner demonstrates foundational knowledge that is cohesive and principled in structure. Typical domain-specific problems become familiar and the learner demonstrates both surface level and deep level strategies. In the final stage of proficiency and expertise, the knowledge base is both wide and deep. Experts engage in problem finding and contribute to new knowledge in the domain.

The Guild Model posits seven stages for expert development. The seven stages are as follows (Data from Hoffman et al. 1995):

Naivette: One who is totally ignorant of the domain.

Novice: Someone who is new.

Initiate: A novice who has begun introductory instruction.

Apprentice: Someone who is learning.

Journeyman: An experienced and reliable worker.

Expert: A distinguished or brilliant journeyman.

Master: A journeyman or expert who is qualified to teach those at a lower level.

What Do We Know About Experts and Expertise?

EXPERTS AND EXPERTISE HAVE BEEN extensively studied in numerous areas, including sports, medicine, music, chess, the military, and leadership. Here is what we know about experts and expertise (Data from Clark 2008).

- Expertise requires practice, often years of practice. For some disciplines, an acceptable level of performance may be relatively easy and relatively quick, perhaps months to a few years. High-level expertise generally takes at least a decade.
- Expertise is domain specific. Being expert at oncology does not qualify one as an expert in pediatrics. Watch Hall of Fame basketball player Charles Barkley swing a golf club to understand this point. Experts outside their realm of expertise solve problems as a novice would.

- Expertise requires deliberate practice. Deliberate practice is specifically tailored to enhance a skill.
- Experts and novices see the world with different eyes. A world-class conductor looks at a musical score differently than a novice.
- Expertise may blind to other approaches and points of view.
- Expertise can be either routine or adaptive. Routine experts solve the typical problems for the domain. Adaptive expertise solves the novel problem.
- Some challenging problems are too large for a single perspective; they requires multiple experts for resolution.

Your Thinking Is a Choice

THE GREEK PHILOSOPHER EPICTETUS WROTE, "People are disturbed not by things, but by the view which they take of them." Or, as Abraham Lincoln observed, "Folks are usually about as happy as they make their minds up to be." Things happen to people; they are reprimanded by a preceptor for being late, or they turn in a substandard assignment. They blame the preceptor or the instructor for their deficiencies in the process. That blame is a choice. Even though the preceptor and instructor may have been less than outstanding, an alternative choice is to accept personal responsibility. You can choose to think someone else is the problem or that you are the problem. The variance in the cascade of behaviors that follow from this choice is significant. One path likely leads to hostility and conflict, whereas the other leads to maturity and personal and professional growth. *In fact, it is this thought—that you are in control of how and what you think—that is the first and most critical step on the path to personal growth.*

Some events, such as a confrontation with an angry patient, can be termed activating events. Because of the event, we respond in a certain way; for example, we lash back or take a negative tone. That is the consequence of the event. The element missing from this scenario, and one that determines our response both emotionally and behaviorally, is the belief about the event. If we believe the patient is a rude, demeaning individual, then we might feel justified in our lashing out at the person. If we believe the patient is a human being worthy of respect and consideration, no matter how he or she behaves, or that the patient is misdirecting his or her frustrations about having significant health concerns, then we are likely to behave with professionalism, compassion, and empathy. This sequence can be reduced to the famous and easily understood formula developed by Albert Ellis:

$$\mathbf{A} \text{ (activating event)} + \mathbf{B} \text{ (belief)} = \mathbf{C} \text{ (consequence)}$$

Effective thinking means that we examine the beliefs we apply to any circumstance to see whether they meet an empirical test (Is there proof that these beliefs are true?), a functional test (Do these beliefs help or make things worse?), and a logical test (Do they meet a test for common sense?). Self-management and personal growth requires that we engage in an internal debate with ourselves, that we dispute with ourselves the validity of our beliefs. If our beliefs are found wanting, then our task is to alter them so that our beliefs, and hence our behaviors, are functional.

Understanding that you control your beliefs in any situation is the beginning of personal and professional growth. As Gandhi observed:

> Your beliefs become your thoughts.
> Your thoughts become your words.
> Your words become your actions.
> Your actions become your habits.
> Your habits become your values.
> Your values become your destiny.

Anyone who has ever come through a significant life event or trauma often recognizes after the fact that, while in the midst of the circumstance, they were thinking "crazy." Personal and professional growth requires an ability to recognize whether we are thinking appropriately about professionalism or whether our thinking is "crazy". Personal and professional growth requires that we be mindful, or aware, of our thinking without being critical or judgmental.

Conclusion

THE CENTRAL IDEA OF THIS chapter is that you are in control of your thinking. Understanding that you control your thinking and then controlling it in the service of your professional obligations is contingent on personal growth in this area. In other words, a person who understands how he or she thinks will be a better professional. Other types of thinking were also discussed, including intuition, judgment, wisdom, practical thinking, and stupidity.

What Do the Practitioners/Others Say?

FOR NEXT CLASS, BE PREPARED to discuss expertise and thinking based on any *one* of the following:

- A discussion with your colleagues, or others, on how they feel or what they know about expertise and thinking.
- An article on expertise and thinking, either from the research literature or any other source.
- A movie, television program, or YouTube video about expertise and thinking.
- A book on expertise and thinking (literary, historical, psychological, or any other source).

Personal Learning Plan: Thinking and Cognition

USE THE FOLLOWING GUIDE TO develop a personal and professional growth project.

What prompted you to develop this plan?	
What is the general area for improvement?	
What is the specific issue for improvement?	
Why is this important to you?	
How do you generally act in these areas?	
What are your goals?	
What strategies are required?	
Who/what is necessary to meet your goals with this strategy?	
How will you measure success/failure with this effort?	
How will you reflect and capture the lesson from this effort that can be generalized to other circumstances?	

The Students: Personal and Professional Issues

BASED ON THE DESCRIPTION OF each student at the beginning of the chapter, what are the personal and professional issues (either immediately or in the future) confronting each student? Consider whether they are linked and, if so, how. Finally, what would you recommend to each student to resolve these issues?

Dana S.

Personal Issues

Professional Issues

Are They Linked? Will the Personal Issues Impact Professional Behavior?

Recommendations

Ivan T.

Personal Issues

Professional Issues

Are They Linked? Will the Personal Issues Impact Professional Behavior?

Recommendations

Niki M.

Personal Issues

Professional Issues

Are They Linked? Will the Personal Issues Impact Professional Behavior?

Recommendations

Ryan P.

Personal Issues

Professional Issues

Are They Linked? Will the Personal Issues Impact Professional Behavior?

Recommendations

Exercises

Six Hat Thinking: A Tool to Help You Think

Edward De Bono (1999) developed the Six Hat Thinking Method. It is a way of looking at a problem from multiple perspectives, but only one at a time. Simplifying the thinking about problems eliminates confusion and helps clarify potential choices. With the Six Hat Thinking Method, only one thing is done at a time.

White Hat Thinking: White hat thinking is to mimic the computer. A computer is neutral. It does not interpret or offer shades of meaning. It is an instrument that deals in facts and information. White hat thinking is objective and analytical. White hat thinking separates information into tiers—that which is proven and absolutely true and that which is believed to be true but is not yet verified. White hat thinking excludes intuition, hunch, and choices based on experience.

Red Hat Thinking: Red hat thinking is about emotion and feeling. It is the opposite of white hat thinking. Ultimately, all decisions are emotional. White hat (analytical) thinking provides a thinking map. In the end, our values and emotions determine the route we take. There is no need to justify an emotion; we just feel that way. Red hat thinking accounts for intuition and hunches. Red hat thinking accounts for deep emotions that might color our choices, such as fear, anger, and jealousy, as well as transient emotions that occur while working through the problem.

Black Hat Thinking: Black hat thinking is the hat of caution. It is not balanced. It is a conscious attempt to consider everything that might go wrong. Black hat thinking is risk assessment—an assessment of the future consequences of a decision taken. Black hat thinking is the most important hat. Its overuse must be guarded against. It is easier to be negative than constructive.

Yellow Hat Thinking: Yellow hat thinking is the opposite of black hat thinking; it is positive and optimistic without being delusional or being a Pollyanna. Yellow hat thinking is a search for value and benefit in our actions that is grounded in logic and analysis. Yellow hat thinking is about visions and dreams.

Green Hat Thinking: Green hat thinking is about new ideas, perceptions, change, and creativity. Green hat thinking attempts to go beyond the known and the obvious in pursuit of a new and better way of doing things.

Blue Hat Thinking: Blue hat thinking is about control, about orchestrating which type of thinking is appropriate at what stage of the process. It is thinking about the type of thinking a problem requires. Blue hat thinking indicates we have spent enough time examining the negative aspects of this problem, and it is now time to examine the benefits to be gained from our choice.

Note the idea in Blue Hat Thinking about controlling how we think. It is critical to understand that you, and only you, control your thinking. As with emotional intelligence, where it is incorrect to say that someone made you feel a certain way, no one makes you think the way you do. If you always think negatively about practice, that is your choice.

Use the Six Hat Thinking Method to work through decisions you may be facing regarding school, career, or personal issues.

Thinking and Professionalism

1. Examine the table below. The point is to surface our thinking about professionalism and its underlying psychology. In other words, what do you believe about personal accountability as a professional? For example, are you motivated to act professionally because of the ultimate financial rewards or because you believe money it is your professional duty?

Beliefs	Professionalism Model	Psychology of Professionalism
	Accountability	Sensitivity
	Altruism	Motivation
	Duty, Honor, Integrity	Judgment
	Excellence	Implementation
	Respect for Others	

2. Record your beliefs in the column provided.

Self-Talk

Self-talk is the voice in our head. If after an argument with someone you go over in your own mind what each of you said and think about what you should have said, you are engaging in self-talk. For the next 5 minutes, listen to the voice in your head. What are you saying to yourself? This self-talk is you "thinking out loud" to yourself and captures an element of your thinking.

Mindfulness

Mindfulness is open and active engagement in aspects of our thinking and feeling in a nonjudgmental way. For some, it is a practice in meditation. For the next several days, try and be mindful of what is going to happen at your job or school. Record your observations in a journal to capture your thought process.

1. Write a one-page executive summary of the chapter.
2. Review the mind map from the opening of the chapter. Would you change anything following reading the chapter?

What's Important to You in the Chapter?

WITH SEVERAL OF YOUR CLASSMATES, discuss the idea or ideas that are most likely to effect change in your values, attitudes, or behaviors. Be succinct. Write no more than two sentences.

References

Baltes, P. B., and Staudinger, U. M. (2000). Wisdom: A metaheuristic (pragmatic) to orchestrate mind and virtue toward excellence. *American Psychologist.* 55, 122–136.

Clark, R. C. (2008). *Building Expertise.* San Francisco, CA: Pfeiffer.

Dane, E., and Pratt, M. G. (2009). Conceptualizing and measuring intuition: A review of recent trends. *International Review of Industrial and Organizational Psychology.* 24, 1–40.

De Bono, E. (1994). *De Bono's Thinking Course.* New York: Facts of File.

De Bono, E. (1999). *Six Thinking Hats.* New York: Back Bay Books.

Friday P. J. (1999). *Friday's Laws: How to Become Normal When You're Not and How to Stay Normal When You Are.* Pittsburgh, PA: Bradley Oak Publications.

Greenhalgh, T. (2002). Intuition and evidence—Uneasy bedfellows. *British Journal of General Practice.* 52 (478), 394–400.

Hammond, J. S., Keeney, R. L., and Raiffa, H. (2006). The hidden traps in decision making. *Harvard Business Review.* January, 118–126.

Hastie, R., and Dawes, R. M. (2001). *Rational Choice in an Uncertain World.* Thousand Oaks, CA: Sage Publications.

Hoffman, R. R., Shadbolt, N. R., Burton, A. M., and Klein, G. (1995). Eliciting knowledge from experts: A methodological analysis. *Organizational Behavior and Human Decision Processes.* 62 (2), 129–158.

Moldoveanu, M., and Langer, E. (2002). When "stupid" is smarter than we are. In *Why Smart People Can Be So Stupid.* R. J. Sternber, ed. New Haven, CT: Yale University Press.

Sternberg, R. (1998). A balance theory of wisdom. *Review of General Psychology.* 2 (4), 347–365.

Welles, J. F. (1991). *The Story of Stupidity.* Orient, NY: Mount Pleasant Press.

Suggested Readings

Albrecht, S. (2009). Evidence-based medicine in pharmacy practice. *US Pharmacist.* 34 (10), 14–18.

Alexander, P. A. (2003). The development of expertise: The journey from acclimation to proficiency. *Educational Researcher.* 32 (8), 10–14.

Ardelt, M. (2004). Wisdom as expert knowledge system: A critical review of a contemporary operationalization of an ancient concept. *Human Development.* 47, 257–285.

Bornstein, B. H., and Emler, A. C. (2001). Rationality in medical decision making: a review of the literature on doctors' decision-making biases. *Journal of Evaluation in Clinical Practice.* 7 (2), 97–107.

Ericsson, K. A., Charness, N., Feltovich, P. J., and Hoffman, R. R. (2006). *The Cambridge Handbook of Expertise and Expert Performance.* Cambridge, United Kingdom: Cambridge University Press.

Ericsson, K. A., and Charness, N. (1994). Expert performance. *American Psychologist.* 49 (8), 725–747.

Ericsson, K. A., Whyte, J., and Ward, P. (2007). Expert performance in nursing. *Advances in Nursing Science*. 30 (1), 58–71.

Farrington-Darby, T., and Wilson, J. R. (2006). The nature of expertise: A review. *Applied Ergonomics*. 37, 17–32

Fox, C. (1997). A confirmatory factor analysis of the structure of tacit knowledge in nursing. *Journal of Nursing Education*. 36 (10), 459–466.

King, L., and Appleton, J. V. (1997). Intuition: A critical review of the research and rhetoric. *Journal of Advanced Nursing*. 26, 194–202.

Mockler, R. J., and Dologite, D. G. (1999). Learning how to learn: Nurturing professional growth through cognitive mapping. *New England Journal of Entrepreneurship*. 2 (2), 65–80.

Nagelkerk, J. (2001). *Diagnostic Reasoning*. Philadelphia, PA: Saunders.

Patel, V. L., Arocha, J. F., and Kaufman, D. R. (1999). Expertise and tacit knowledge in medicine. In *Tacit Knowledge in Professional Practice*. R. J. Sternberg and J. A. Horvath, eds. New York: Routledge.

Patel, V. L., Kaufman, D. R., and Magder, S. A. (1996). The acquisition of medical expertise in complex dynamic environments. In *The Road to Excellence*. K. A. Ericsson, ed. Mahwah, NJ: Lawrence Erlbaum Associates.

Quirk, M. (2006). *Intuition and Metacognition in Medical Education*. New York: Spring Publishing Co.

Schmidt, H. G., and Boshuizen, P. A. (1993). On acquiring expertise in medicine. *Educational Psychology Review*. 5 (3), 205–221.

Tversky, A., and Khaneman, D. (1974). Judgment under uncertainty: Heuristics and biases. *Science*. 185, 1124–1131.

Wagner, R. K., and Sternberg, R. J. (1985). Practical intelligence in real-world pursuits: The role of tacit knowledge. *Journal of Personality and Psychology*. 49 (2), 436–458.

Millennials and Working Across Generations

Preassessment: Millennials

Mind Mapping

*Consider the phrase displayed on the page. For this phrase, without thinking or editing, write down the ideas, concepts, examples, contradictions, and theories that come to mind. Do not array them in any systematic or orderly manner. Scatter them about the page. Now, draw lines between your additions, indicating that there is a relationship between the terms. If something causes something else, indicate this with an arrow. Relationships may be reciprocal, meaning both cause each other, requiring arrows at both ends. Indicate the strength of the relationships by darkening and thickening the lines; stronger relationships have darker and thicker lines. **Most important: There is no right answer. Do not compare with your classmates.** What you have is a mind map, your mental representation of these topics. Review to determine if anything has changed following this section.*

Rights of a Student

The Students

I

DANA S. HATED TO WRITE papers. Even though the writing itself was private, Dana knew she would be revealing something of what she thought. She also knew the particular assignment she was working on required being prepared to discuss the paper informally in class. She knew how it would work. The instructor would start at the front of the room and ask for a brief synopsis of the paper and then begin a series of probing questions. Dana had to admit that the questions were relatively gentle and usually not challenging, but she hated to talk in class. Some of her classmates had tried to draw her into a discussion of the politics related to health care after class last week. She believed some of the comments were foolish; she knew she had better ideas. She left once the conversation got heated. There was one student in the discussion who Dana thought was attractive. She wished she would have stayed because she wanted to get to know him better.

Finishing the paper around 1:00 AM a week before it was due, Dana sent it via email to the instructor asking him to review it for comments. About 4 days later, the instructor responded with a curt reply that he would not review the paper prior to grading. He attached the requirements for the assignment and told Dana to assess her own work relative to the standards. Dana was upset because it took so long for a response and because he wouldn't review the paper. For the tuition she was paying, Dana believed she deserved an immediate response and a review. Dana was considering calling her mother to ask for her help and to have her call the instructor, the chairman of his department, and the dean of the school.

II

Ivan T. had only had two semesters left before graduation. He couldn't believe it. His average for an important clinical course was 69.1. He missed a passing grade by 0.4 point. Now he would have to retake the course. Unless he could find the points somewhere else, his graduation would be delayed. Ivan calculated that if he had to delay graduation for a year he would lose approximately $100,000 in salary and have to borrow another $10,000 for expenses for that year, not to mention the extra tuition for the course.

If Ivan were honest with himself, he would have to admit that he had been warned. In meetings with the instructor and the faculty advisor, when he discussed his work schedule and his need for money to support his apartment and a planned Christmas excursion to Europe, they told him he needed to review his priorities. His mother had also warned him.

In fact, Ivan's average for the course was 66.1, but the instructor had added a 3.0-point curve to all of the students' scores. Ivan was considering his negotiation strategy with the instructor. His first appeal would be based on sympathy and a recounting of his personal story and his profound desire to help his mother who had struggled to raise him as a single mother. If that didn't work, he would threaten the instructor (who was foreign born) with a lawsuit claiming incompetence and discrimination. He thought the discrimination approach might work because he and the instructor had often clashed when having health policy discussions. He also had told the instructor in private that he would never use the ideas they were discussing in class in practice. Ivan told the instructor he planned to go into managed care and that the clinical minutiae of the course were not relevant to him. This was an exaggeration; Ivan didn't really know what he wanted to do.

III

Niki M. looked over the syllabus and calculated how much time she needed to devote to this course. It was labeled as writing intensive, which meant a single small paper was due at mid-term and a larger paper was due at the end of the semester. For her, this requirement would be a breeze. She was a naturally gifted writer, and her skills had been honed in her undergraduate program. After the first night of class, Niki had the course measured. She seriously considered cutting all of the classes with the exception of those when the papers were due. She would synthesize the material on her own. Although the school did not have a formal attendance policy, she knew that this professor would pick up on her absence.

She decided she would use the class time for reviewing her other notes. She would only "tune in" to the lecture and discussion when she sensed something that might be relevant for the paper was brought up. So far, after 2 weeks, nothing that was not in the handouts and readings had been discussed.

Last week in class, Niki's instructor looked over Niki's shoulder at her computer. She asked Niki to put it away. Niki put the computer away slowly, with exaggeration and attitude. Niki was so incensed by the public censure that she left the class 10 minutes early. When Niki got home, an email was already waiting for her requesting that she meet with the instructor before class next week. Niki thought the instructor should be happy she came to class. Niki was certain the instructor did not know how tight her schedule was with school, a child, and a job.

Niki now found herself outside the instructor's door. She was still upset about last week. Niki was not sure what she was going to say.

IV

Ryan P. really loved hockey, and the playoffs had begun. A member of Ryan's class group (who were all in their 20s) had scheduled that night, the night of a hockey playoff game, to have a meeting regarding their group presentation. All five members of the group met at a local pub next to campus to work on the project. As they sat down, the rest of the group discussed movies and artists that Ryan had no clue about. Ryan generally liked all the members of the group. He found them interesting and considered their behaviors and attitudes as a window on what his daughter would be like next year when she went to college. Ryan had allocated an hour for the session to be certain to make the opening of the hockey game.

None of the students came prepared. They had the instructions for the project from the instructor, but no one had done their preparation. The first 15 minutes of the meeting were taken up with emails, texting, and complaints about how the instructor expected way too much of them. Also, they complained that the project was boring; they weren't challenged. The students felt it should be enough to come to class and take the tests. This project hardly seemed relevant to them. Now, 30 minutes had passed with no productive work. One of the students complained that when she discussed their ideas with the instructor, the instructor hadn't been supportive enough. The instructor made the comment that although she appreciated the effort, she would only grade on their performance. Now there was only 15 minutes left, and Ryan was getting frustrated—he wanted to make the start of the game.

✦ LEARNING OBJECTIVES

- Describe generational theory.
- Describe some of the characteristics of a Millennial.
- List and discuss the perceived orientation of Millennials.
- Discus the research findings on Millennials.
- Discuss aspects of working across generations.

✦ KEY TERMS

- Generational theory
- Millennial

How Do I View This Chapter?

IF YOU ARE A MILLENNIAL, the way to view this chapter is as a mirror, reflecting back to you what is being written and claimed about you and your generational cohort. Some of it is true of the majority of people characterized as **Millennials**. Some claims apply to a relatively few individuals. Nevertheless, the assumptions others make about you and people your age help explain what they think about you, their expectations for you, and how they treat you. In reading this chapter, consider whether the generational attributes that follow are true for you and, if so, to what degree. Also consider whether the attributes are functional for you now and for your future career. Finally, consider whether the stereotypes of an entire generation of over 75 million people are accurate.

What Is Generational Theory?

GENERATIONAL THEORY SUGGESTS THAT PEOPLE of approximately the same age exhibit similar attitudes, behaviors, and beliefs as a result of having matured at the same time and been subject to the same influences. Different generations of workers/practitioners are assumed to differ in their values related to work, work relationships, communication, incentives, attitudes toward leadership, commitment to the organization, how they learn, and career progression. Generally those influences are family, education, morality, peers, spirituality, and culture. All generations are influenced by war, social movements, economics, and technological advances. The impact varies, however, based on the stage in life. Each generation has a collective memory of a shared past. Where were you when Pearl Harbor was attacked, when Kennedy was shot, when Reagan was shot, or when Michael Jackson died? Events experienced as a person comes of age are imprinted on them and serve as templates for their attitudes and behaviors for the rest of their lives.

Generational Descriptions

THE FOLLOWING TABLE SUMMARIZES THE key historical events that have impacted the last four generations and the traits associated with that generation.

	Millennials	Generation Xers	Baby Boomers	Traditionalists
Time Span	1980–2001	1965–1979	1946–1964	1925–1945
Current residents, U.S. Census Bureau estimate	92 million	62 million	78.3 million	38.6 million
Key historical events	Columbine September 11 attack Enron War in Iraq, Afghanistan Hurricane Katrina	AIDS epidemic Challenger catastrophe Fall of Berlin Wall Oklahoma City bombings Clinton scandal	Vietnam War John F. Kennedy, Robert Kennedy, and Martin Luther King assassinations First man on moon Kent State shootings Watergate	Great Depression Pearl Harbor World War II Korean War Cold War Cuban Missile Crisis

(continues)

	Millennials	Generation Xers	Baby Boomers	Traditionalists
Time Span	1980–2001	1965–1979	1946–1964	1925–1945
Traits	Entitled Optimistic Civic minded Close parental involvement Work–life balance Impatient Multitask Team oriented	Self-reliant Adaptable Cynical Distrust authority Resourceful Entrepre-neurial Technologi-cally savvy	Workaholic Idealistic Competitive Loyal Materialistic Seeking personal fulfillment Values titles and corner office	Patriotic Dependable Conformist Respect authority Rigid Socially and financially Conservative Work ethic

Data from Alsop, R. (2008). *The Trophy Kids Grow Up*. San Francisco, CA: Jossey-Bass.

What Is a Millennial?

DEMOGRAPHICALLY, MILLENNIALS ARE INDIVIDUALS BORN between approximately 1980 and 2000. There are about 90 million people in this cohort in the United States, approximately a quarter of the population. The Millennial generation is equivalent in size to the Baby Boomer generation, those born from 1946 to 1964. Millennials have been described as trophy kids who are high maintenance and needy. As children, they received gold stars for showing up and given trophies for finishing ninth. Rather than being trained by their parents, they were nurtured. They were special. They were sheltered. They have close relationships with their parents who take an active part in their lives. They are narcissistic with a sense of entitlement. Many still live at home. Many delay the normal progressions of adulthood. They are team oriented. Faculty and instructors may see them as whiny, needy, seeking instant gratification, and grade oriented.

The May 20, 2013, cover of *Time* magazine portrayed a reclining girl taking a picture of herself with an iPhone under the title: "The ME ME ME

Generation." This is how this generation is thought of by many. Most relevant to you is the fact that many of the people hiring Millennials, most likely to be Baby Boomers or Gen X, think of you this way. Two distinct characterizations of millennials from that issue of *Time* follow. They are stereotypes. They contain elements of the truth, but they are not the complete truth.

> Here's the cold, hard data: The incidence of narcissistic personality disorder is nearly three times as high for people in their 20s as for the generation that's now 65 or older, according to the National Institutes of Health: 58% more college students scored higher on a narcissism scale in 2009 than in 1982. Millennials got so many participation trophies growing up that a recent study showed that 40% believe they should be promoted every two years, regardless of performance. They are fame obsessed: three times as many middle school girls want to grow up to be a personal assistant to a famous person as want to be a Senator, according to a 2007 survey; four times as many would pick the assistant job over CEO of a major corporation. They're so convinced of their own greatness that the National Study of Youth and Religion found the guiding morality of 60% of millennials in any situation is that they'll just be able to feel what is right. Their development is stunted: more people ages 18 to 29 live with their parents than with a spouse, according to the 2012 Clark University Poll of Emerging Adults. And they are lazy. In 1992, the nonprofit Families and Work Institute reported that 80% of people under 23 wanted one day to have a job with greater responsibility; 10 years later, only 60% did. (Stein 2013, p. 28)

So here's a more rounded picture of millennials than the one I started with. All of which I have data for. They're earnest and optimistic. They embrace the system. They are pragmatic idealists, tinkerers more than dreamers, life hackers. Their world is so flat that they have no leaders, which is why revolutions like Occupy Wall Street to Tahrir Square have even less chance than previous rebellions. They want constant approval—they post photos from the dressing room as they try on clothes. The have massive fear of missing out and an acronym for everything (including FOMO). They're celebrity obsessed but don't respectfully idolize celebrities from a distance. (Thus *Us* magazine's "They're just like us!" which consists of paparazzi shots of famous people doing everyday things.) They're not into going to church, even though they believe in God, because they don't identify with big institutions: one-third of adults under 30, the highest percentage ever, are religiously unaffiliated. They want new experiences, which are more important to them than material goods. They are cool and reserved and not all that passionate. They are informed but inactive: they hate Joseph Kony but aren't going to do anything about Joseph Kony. They are probusiness. They're financially responsible; although student loans have hit record highs, they have less household and credit-card debt than any previous generation on record—which, admittedly, isn't that hard when you are living at home and using your parent's credit card. They love their phones but hate talking on them. (Stein 2013, p. 34)

Perceived Orientation of Millennials

OVER 2 YEARS, RESEARCHERS ESPINOZA, Ukleja, and Rusch (2010) interviewed hundreds of managers and employees in various work environments. From that effort they recognized nine perceived orientations of Millennials. These orientations are how managers perceive millennial employees. When Millennials themselves were asked for their reactions to these perceptions, they confirmed their validity. In other words, both managers and Millennials themselves agree on a composite picture of Millennial orientations. These orientations are termed "points of tension" between managers and Millennial employees. The nine orientations are as follows (Data from Espinoza, Ukleja, and Rusch 2010):

Autonomous: Millennials want to do what they want when they want, to have the schedule they want, and to not be micromanaged. As long as they complete the work, Millennials do not want to conform to standard procedures. The intrinsic value underlying the orientation is work–life balance.

Entitled: Millennials believe they deserve to be recognized and rewarded. They want a guarantee for their performance, not just an opportunity. They want to move up quickly. The intrinsic value underlying the orientation is reward.

Imaginative: Millennials have great imaginations and a unique way of looking at things. Imagination can distract from participation in ordered processes. The intrinsic value underlying the orientation is self–expression.

Self-Absorbed: Millennials are concerned with themselves and about how they are treated, not how they treat others. Millennials are focused on their need for trust, encouragement, and praise. The intrinsic value underlying the orientation is attention.

Defensive: Millennials want to be told when they are doing well not when they are deficient. They are often angry and defensive and shift responsibility when confronted with inadequate performance. The intrinsic value underlying the orientation is achievement.

Abrasive: Millennial style of communication is curt, perhaps due to technology. They seem to lack some of the social graces. It comes across as disrespectful. The intrinsic value underlying the orientation is informality.

Myopic: Millennials are internally focused and have difficulty understanding how others and the organization are impacted. Cause and effect escapes them. The intrinsic value underlying the orientation is simplicity.

Unfocused: Millennials have a hard time staying focused on tasks and often do not pay attention to detail. The intrinsic value underlying the orientation is multitasking.

Indifferent: Millennials are perceived as careless, apathetic, or lacking commitment. The intrinsic value underlying the orientation is meaning.

Millennials: The Empirical Evidence

MUCH THAT IS WRITTEN ABOUT Millennials is based on anecdotal accounts from human resources professionals and current supervisors. Their comments are impressions based on a limited number of cases. As such, the validity of these impressions may be questionable. The conclusions discussed below are included because there is empirical support for those conclusions, although it may not be overwhelming. Generally, the attempt has been to avoid such academic reviews. However, in this case, it is the point—the contrast between anecdote and empirical findings.

Narcissism is a psychological term. Common synonyms for it include arrogance, conceit, vanity, grandiosity, and self-centeredness. Narcissists have unwarranted estimates of their worth and capabilities. Narcissists believe they are special, entitled, and unique. The extremes of this pattern of behavior warrant a clinical diagnosis of narcissistic personality disorder (NPD). The focus here is on the narcissistic personality as opposed to the pathological diagnosis of NPD. Narcissism is argued to develop from excessive and indulgent parenting that focuses on self-esteem and making a child feel special, devoid of accurate feedback regarding performance, along with cultural influences that worship celebrity, self-promotion, and the cult of "we are all special."

Twenge et.al. (2008) reviewed studies of over 16,000 college students and concluded that there is a definite upswing in narcissism. Putting this in perspective, the increase in narcissism over the last few decades is the equivalent in the increase in obesity in the country over the same time period. In another study of over 1.4 million people, primarily college students, from the 1930s to the present (Twenge and Campbell 2008), it was found that:

- The need for social approval is down.
- Self-esteem and narcissism are up.
- Locus of control is more external (attributing the control of events to external forces in the environment).
- Anxiety and depression are up.
- Women are more assertive and agentic.

Small differences in the centrality of work have been found, with it being lower for younger generations than for older ones (Smola and Sutton 2002; Twenge et al. 2010).

The stereotype is that millennials work less than older generations. In fact, the Families and Work Institute (2005) found that there is no difference in the hours worked for Generation Xers and Millennials at the same age. Staff and Schulenberg (2010) found that the generations are similar in their work patterns during high school, and Millennials do not work less than Baby Boomers or Xers at the same age.

Compared to other generations, Millennials have higher rates of obesity and are less fit than Baby Boomers and Xers at the same age (Wang et al. 2008).

Millennials may not be as academically prepared as previous generations. At the end of high school, Millennials did not know substantially more than previous generations at the same age (Deal, Altman, and Rogelberg 2010).

It is hypothesized for medical students that because of their perfectionism, Millennials will be higher than Gen Xers on the need for achievement;

because of their affinity for teams, Millennials will be higher than Gen Xers on their need for affiliation; and because of their desire to work in teams and solve problems, Millennials will be higher on the need for power than Gen Xers. The findings are that Millennials score higher on the need for achievement and the need for affiliation than Gen Xers (Borges et al. 2010)

Working Across Generations

A GRADUATING STUDENT IS LIKELY TO work with members from the Silent Generation, Baby Boomers, Gen Xers, and Millennials. More than likely, their superiors will be Baby Boomers or Gen Xers. Understanding how to work across generations and for superiors of a different generation is important, because negotiating this aspect of work will determine your career trajectory. It is a fact that, for the time being, power resides with people older than you.

First, you need to accept that you are not likely to change your personality, and neither is your superior. Personality and behavioral tendencies are relatively fixed for most people. Change is only likely to occur following a significant event. Thus, thinking that problems would go away if the other person would only change and be somebody different is not going to happen. Learn to work with people as they are.

Second, understand your work relationship with your boss. You are involved in a mutually dependent relationship between two fallible human beings. Each of you has strengths, weaknesses, talents, goals, problems, and pressures. Your superiors are not all powerful; they are dependent on you, just as you are dependent on them. You need to understand what your superiors' issues are, their work style, and the issues they may have with their superiors.

Third, just as you would ask your superiors to understand your circumstances, your values, and the events that shaped your world, it is only fair to ask you to consider the same things for your superiors. What are their values? What shaped their world? Like you, your superiors will find it difficult to get outside their own skin. In other words, it is difficult for them, just like it is difficult for you, to accurately assess their own traits, expectations, and behaviors. Try to understand what it is like to be a Gen Xer or a Baby Boomer. As with you, caution in accepting generational stereotypes as universal is warranted.

"When you boil it down, Millennials expect special attention because they believe they are special. Their parents have told them, their schools have told them, television has told them. Now it's management's turn" (Espinoza, Ukleja, and Rusch 2010, p. 84). The Baby Boomer or Gen Xer generations may think of their own son or daughter as special, but they most likely will not see you as special in a work context. To expect or demand special treatment at work is to sabotage your career.

Finally, work is an exchange. The reason you are employed and the justification for your salary is the fact that you add economic value in excess of the cost of your salary. You are there to solve problems for the company. You are neither entitled to nor guaranteed a job or a successful career. The only job security is in efficiently and effectively meeting the demands of the consumer marketplace. Despite what you might think, everyone in the company has this same standard to meet; everyone from CEO to housekeeping is in the consumer satisfaction business. As Sam Walton noted, "There is only one boss. The customer. And he can fire everybody in the company from the chairman on down, simply by spending his money somewhere else." Make no mistake: a company will cut your hours, close your department, or close your store if the economics warrant. Mark Twain captured this perspective by declaring, "Don't go around saying the world owes you a living; the world owes you nothing; it was here first."

Given an understanding of this reality, your part of the work exchange is to get what you want from the company; it is how you define winning the work game. Do not feel guilty about this. Your aspiration may be to rise to the upper echelons of the organization by age 40, have a stable job in a facility close to your family, or go part time in 5–10 years while you raise your family. Your objective is yours alone. If a specific practice setting or organization will not let you accomplish your goals, then it is time to move.

"In our opinion many of the Millennials who are promoted into management get the invite because they appear different from their peers—more mature. They take an interest in their superiors and are able to reach up and make a connection. Therefore, they draw attention and favor of the older generations. We found that approximately one in five Millennials take the initiative to connect with their superiors" (Espinoza, Ukleja, and Rusch 2010, p. 21). This is good advice. Your relationship with your superiors is yours—and yours alone. You have to manage that relationship, like any other, to get what you want.

Conclusion

THIS CHAPTER PRESENTED A PICTURE of the Millennial generation, both anecdotal and empirical. The idea of different generations being influenced by different circumstances was presented as well as suggestions for working across generations.

What Do the Practitioners/Others Say?

FOR NEXT CLASS, BE PREPARED to discuss perspectives on the Millennials based on any *one* of the following:

- A discussion with your colleagues, or others, on how they feel and what they know about Millennials.
- An article on Millennials either from the research literature or any other source.
- A movie, television program, or YouTube video about Millennials.
- A book on Millennials (literary, historical, psychological, or any other source).

Personal Learning Plan: Millennials

USE THE FOLLOWING GUIDE TO develop a personal and professional growth project.

What prompted you to develop this plan?	
What is the general area for improvement?	
What is the specific issue for improvement?	
Why is this important to you?	
How do you generally act in these areas?	
What are your goals?	
What strategies are required?	
Who/what is necessary to meet your goals with this strategy?	
How will you measure success/failure with this effort?	
How will you reflect and capture the lesson from this effort that can be generalized to other circumstances?	

The Students: Personal and Professional Issues

BASED ON THE DESCRIPTION OF each student at the beginning of the chapter, what are the personal and professional issues (either immediately or in the future) confronting each student? Consider whether they are linked and, if so, how. Finally, what would you recommend to each student to resolve these issues?

Dana S.

Personal Issues

Professional Issues

Are They Linked? Will the Personal Issues Impact Professional Behavior?

Recommendations

Ivan T.

Personal Issues

Professional Issues

Are They Linked? Will the Personal Issues Impact Professional Behavior?

Recommendations

Niki M.

Personal Issues

Professional Issues

Are They Linked? Will the Personal Issues Impact Professional Behavior?

Recommendations

Ryan P.

Personal Issues

Professional Issues

Are They Linked? Will the Personal Issues Impact Professional Behavior?

Recommendations

Exercises

Generational Views

In your family, consider your parents' and grandparents' attitudes toward:

Money

Careers

Work

Family

Politics

Diversity

Same-sex marriage

Marijuana

iPhones

The Affordable Care Act

Organized religion

Where did these attitudes come from? What events shaped these attitudes?

Perceived Orientations of Millennials and Professionalism

With several of your classmates, discuss whether the following perceived orientations of Millennials are accurate and fair.

Autonomous: Millennials want to do what they want when they want, to have the schedule they want, and to not be micromanaged.

Entitled: Millennials believe they deserve to be recognized and rewarded.

Imaginative: Millennials have great imaginations and a unique way of looking at things.

Self-Absorbed: Millennials are concerned with themselves and about how they are treated, not how they treat others.

Defensive: Millennials want to be told when they are doing well, not when they are deficient. They are often angry and defensive and shift responsibility when confronted with inadequate performance.

Abrasive: Millennial style of communication is curt, perhaps due to technology. They seem to lack some of the social graces. It comes across as disrespectful.

Myopic: Millennials are internally focused and have difficulty understanding how others and the organization are impacted. Cause and effect escapes them.

Unfocused: Millennials have a hard time staying focused on tasks and often do not pay attention to detail.

Indifferent: Millennials are perceived as careless, apathetic, or lacking commitment.

Narcissism Personality Inventory

In each of the following pairs, choose the one that you *most agree* with. Circle your answer. Only mark *one answer* for each attitude pair.

1. A. The thought of ruling the world frightens the hell out of me.

   B. If I ruled the world, it would be a much better place.

2. A. I prefer to blend in with the crowd.

   B. I like to be the center of attention.

3. A. I can live my life any way I want to.

   B. People can't always live their lives in terms of what they want.

4. A. I don't particularly like to show off my body.

   B. I like to show off my body.

5. A. I will never be satisfied until I get all that I deserve.

   B. I will take my satisfactions as they come.

6. A. I am no better or no worse than most people.

   B. I think I am a special person.

7. A. I find it easy to manipulate people.

   B. I don't like it when I find myself manipulating people.

8. A. I try not to be a show-off.

    B. I will usually show off if I get the chance.

9. A. I am much like everybody else.

    B. I am an extraordinary person.

10. A. I like having authority over other people.

    B. I don't mind following orders.

Questions 3, 5, 7, and 10: Give yourself 1 point if you answered A.

Questions 1, 2, 4, 6, 8, and 9: Give yourself 1 point if you answered B.

0–3 points: Low in narcissism.

4–5 points: About the same in narcissism as the average college student.

6–7 points: Above average in narcissism.

8–10 points: Significantly above average in narcissism.

Twenge, J. M., and Campbell, W. K. (2010). *The Narcissism Epidemic.* New York: Free Press.

Millennials and Baby Boomers

Discuss the likely tensions in a work group composed of Millennials and Baby Boomers. What could be done to negate these potential conflicts? Who gets assigned what roles? Can both groups be made happy at the same time, or will their always be issues?

Generation Y (Millennials) and Baby Boomers

Interestingly, the oldest (Baby Boomers) and youngest (Generation Y, Millennials) cohorts at work demand many of the same things. Based on work by Hewlett, Sherbin, and Sumberg (2009), the following portraits of each generation emerge.

Portrait of Generation Y (Millennials)

- 84% profess to be very ambitious
- 45% expect to work for their current employer their entire career
- 78% are comfortable working with people from different backgrounds
- 86% say it is important that their work makes a positive impact on the world

- 48% say having a network of friends at work is very important

Portrait of Baby Boomers

- 42% project they will continue working after age 65
- 46% see themselves as being in the middle of their careers
- 55% are members of external volunteer networks
- 87% say being able to work flexibly is important
- 71% report having elder care responsibilities

Generation Y (Millennials) rate the following six types of rewards as at least as important as compensation (in order of importance):

- High-quality colleagues
- Flexible work arrangements
- Prospects for advancement
- Recognition from one's company or boss
- A steady state of advancement
- Access to new experiences and challenges

Baby Boomers rate the following seven types of rewards as at least as important as compensation (in order of importance):

- High-quality colleagues
- An intellectually stimulating work place
- Autonomy regarding work tasks
- Flexible work arrangements
- Access to new experiences and challenges
- Giving back to the world through work
- Recognition from one's company or boss

1. Write a one page executive summary of the chapter.
2. Review the mind map from the opening of the chapter. Would you change anything following reading the chapter?

What's Important to You in the Chapter?

WITH SEVERAL OF YOUR CLASSMATES, discuss the idea or ideas that are most likely to effect change in your values, attitudes, or behaviors. Be succinct. Write no more than two sentences

References

Alsop, R. (2008). *The Trophy Kids Grow Up*. San Francisco, CA: Jossey-Bass.

Borges, N. J., Manuel, R. S., Elam, C. L., and Jones, B. J. (2010). Differences in motives between Millennial and Generation X medical students. *Medical Education*. 44, 570–576.

Deal, J. J., Altman, D. G., and Rogelberg, S. G. (2010). Millennials at work: What we know and what we need to do (if anything). *Journal of Business Psychology*. 25, 191–199.

Espinoza, C., Ukleja, M., and Rusch, C. (2010). *Managing the Millennials*. Hoboken, NJ: John Wiley & Sons.

Families and Work Institute. (2005). Generations and gender in the workplace. http://familiesandwork.org/site/research/reports/GG-managertips.pdf. Accessed January 14, 2014.

Hewlett, S. A., Sherbin, L., and Sumberg, K. (2009). How Gen Y and Boomers will reshape your agenda. *Harvard Business Review*. July–August, 1–7.

Smola, K. W., and Sutton, C. D. (2002). Generational differences: Revisiting generational work values for the new millennium. *Journal of Organizational Behavior*. 23, 363–382.

Staff, J., and Schulenberg, J. (2010). Millennials and the world of work: Experiences in paid work during adolescence. *Journal of Business and Psychology*. 25, 247–255.

Stein J. The new greatest generation. *Time Magazine*, May 20, 2013, p. 28.

Twenge, J. M., and Campbell, W. K. (2008). Generational differences in psychological traits and their impact on the workforce. *Journal of Managerial Psychology*. 23 (8), 862–877.

Twenge, J. M., and Campbell, W. K. (2010). *The Narcissism Epidemic*. New York: Free Press.

Twenge, J. M., Campbell, S. M., Hoffman, B. J., and Lance, C. E. (2010). Generational differences in work values: Leisure and extrinsic values increasing, social and intrinsic values decreasing. *Journal of Management*. 36, 1117–1142.

Twenge, J. M., Konrath S., Foster, J. D., Campbell, W. K., and Bushman, B. J. (2008). Egos inflating over time: A cross-temporal meta-analysis of the narcissistic personality inventory. *J. of Personality*, 76 (4), 875–901.

Wang, Y., Beydoun, M. A., Liang, L., Caballero, B., and Kumanyika, S. K. (2008). Will all Americans become overweight or obese? Estimating the progression and costs of the U. S. obesity epidemic. *Obesity*. 16, 2323–2330.

Suggested Readings

Gabarro, J. J., and Kotter, J. P. (2005). Managing your boss. *Harvard Business Review*. January, 92–99.

Taylor, P., and Keeter, S. (2010). *Millennials: A Portrait of Generation Next.* Washington, DC: Pew Research Center.

Tulgan, B. (2009). *Not Everyone Gets a Trophy.* San Francisco: CA: Jossey-Bass.

CHAPTER
9

Impressions

Preassessment: Impressions

Mind Mapping

*Consider the phrase displayed on the page. For this term, without thinking or editing, write down the ideas, concepts, examples, contradictions, and theories that come to mind. Do not arrange them in any systematic or orderly manner. Scatter them about the page. Now, draw lines between your additions indicating that there is a relationship between the terms. If something causes something else, indicate this with an arrow. Relationships may be reciprocal, meaning both cause each other, requiring arrows at both ends. Indicate the strength of the relationships by darkening and thickening the lines; stronger relationships have darker and thicker lines. **Most important: There is no right answer. Do not compare with your classmates.** What you have is a mind map, your mental representation of these topics. Review to determine if anything has changed following this section.*

First Impressions

The Students

I

WHEN DANA S. WAS NERVOUS or felt challenged, she tried to make herself small, to shrink into invisibility if possible. Lately, she had been trying to understand why she behaved like this. She thought that she could connect it to an incident when she was a little girl. She had forgotten exactly what she had said, but she remembered that both her mother and father had publicly chastised and embarrassed her for something she had said to their friends. Although she had forgotten the specific comment, she remembered that it was about the arguing and noises she heard coming from their bedroom. When she was extremely nervous, Dana would often cry. The last time this had happened was only 2 years ago. Even in one-on-one situations, if Dana felt challenged, she became nervous and would lose her composure and shut down. Even worse, she would sometimes blush, and not just on her face but also on her neck and chest. When that happened, all she could focus on was the blushing.

Now Dana was preparing for a job interview that she really wanted. What made the preparation worse was that her mother was hovering around offering advice. Not only was her mother trying to insert herself into the preparations, but she was also engaging in some heavy guilt manipulation. Her mother kept asking, "If you take this job, how often will you come home to see me? Will you call me? Are you going to forget about me?" At this point, her mother dropped the big news. Her mother revealed that she and Dana's father were separating and that he had moved out and was going to file divorce papers. Her mother broke down and started to cry. She said he had already moved in with someone else. He told her he had only been waiting for Dana to graduate. Dana thought to herself, "It has always been about you. I never have been in the spotlight."

II

Ivan T. was extremely handsome. He had impeccable taste in clothes and an athletic body that was model slim and buffed. He worked at looking good. When things were bad or he was stressed, Ivan used the gym as a release. Ivan was nutritionally savvy and diligent. He knew his daily calorie, fat, protein, and carbohydrate intake. He was a regular at the health food store in search of ever better supplements. When everything around Ivan had been chaotic, the one thing he could control was what went into his mouth. In fact, Ivan often considered leveraging his degree into graduate work focusing on the mind–body connection and health, the nutritional patterns and requirements of elite athletes, or the performance psychology of elite athletes.

He followed the various men's magazines looking for trends and fashionable colors. He knew how clothes should be cut and how they should fit. He favored a European cut and slightly offbeat colors. Ivan sensed that this orientation might have had something to do with the fact that his entire adolescence and early adulthood had been tinged with depression, sadness, rejection, cancer, and death and dying. For Ivan, the clothes were an affirmation of life, a marker that this troubled past was over.

Ivan knew what the acceptable "uniform" was for a job interview—dark suit, white shirt, conservative tie, and lace-up dress shoes. Ivan hated the thought of this. He hated having to spend the money on these clothes, but he did. Now, as he was dressing for the interview, rather than being excited by the prospect of a job with one of the largest corporations in the industry, he had a feeling of a coffin being closed. As he walked out the door, Ivan wondered how the interview would go.

III

Besides her considerable intellect, Niki M. had two other outstanding gifts. The first was her athleticism. It had paid for her undergraduate degree. The second was her quick wit. It was a natural gift; in a conversation, she could turn a question back on itself, find the inconsistency in an argument, or highlight the obvious stupidity in someone's statement. She had learned this style at the family dinner table. If you weren't witty and quick, nobody paid attention to you. Her father could be argumentative. For him, it was just conversation, nothing personal. Plus, Niki was funny. Her humor just spilled out. Sometimes she just had to go for the joke, even though it might be inappropriate in the context.

Niki's athleticism and quick wit were now a problem. As an athlete, she had never really learned or cared for some of the attributes that society thought of as feminine. Niki was not petite, dainty, or demure. She did not cater to other people's needs. Competitiveness and aggressiveness were assets on the playing field. She did not defer if she believed somebody was wrong. While some girls were perfecting the art of shopping, dressing well, and ingratiating themselves, Niki was wearing sweats, running, and lifting.

Niki had decided to forego clinical practice and was interviewing with consulting firms that serviced the industry. Niki passed the first interview easily. She knew that this particular firm exhibited at various industry conventions where social sophistication was required. She had been invited for a second interview, this time with two senior partners and their wives at an expensive restaurant downtown. Niki wondered what to wear, what to say, and even if she should go. She really wanted this job.

IV

Ryan P. knew how to dress, present himself, make small talk, look people in the eye, shake hands firmly, make people feel important, and get people to talk about themselves. On first meeting, Ryan would appear confident, in control, and as someone capable of taking care of himself and any situation he might encounter. In the corporate world he came from, Ryan was confident, polished, and capable.

If only this was also true in his current situation. Class was a struggle. All the memorization in the program was a struggle. At home, Ryan sensed his family disintegrating. One daughter was leaving for college, the other was pulling away as she moved through her adolescence, and his wife was reestablishing a career outside the home. Ryan felt his world was lacking stability. Because of the way he presented himself, instructors and faculty assumed Ryan had things under control. In any laboratory or clinical exercise, his instructors did not focus on him. They assumed Ryan was "getting it." Sometimes Ryan needed their help, but he just couldn't bring himself to ask for it. He didn't know why, but he would never ask for extra attention. He would go home and try to work out any problems himself, which could be isolating and time consuming.

✸ LEARNING OBJECTIVES

- Discuss creating a first impression.
- Discuss how to establish credibility.
- Discuss the precautions related to social media.
- Discuss real professionalism.

✸ KEY TERMS

- Credibility
- Exemplification
- Ingratiation
- Intimidation
- Self-promotion
- Supplication

"Professionalism is not a label you give yourself—it's a description you hope others will apply to you."

Maister 2000, p. 17

First Impressions

MUCH OF THE TYPICAL DISCUSSION on professionalism focuses on presentation. How does one look? Do he speak appropriately? Is her communication (verbal and written) appropriate? Does he act accordingly? Does she arrive on time? This approach is termed impression management, which is the conscious and unconscious effort by an individual to influence other people's perceptions of them. It is about constructing an image—a professional image. Please note that image must be crafted to the context. One environment may require business attire, while another requires clothes for the field. A professional image has value for the individual. Being noted by others as professional begets influence and translates into power. That influence and power can be used to advance career and organizational objectives and can also translate into improved patient care and outcomes. Professional demeanor is a currency. It has to be acquired.

We have complete control over how we present ourselves, including how we dress, our facial expressions, our posture and physical presence, our hairstyles, and so on. What we do not control is the perceptions others have of us. Others view us through filters, lenses, and influences that may distort their perceptions. Those filters include meta programs—the way people think and their approach to thinking. Some people value substance over style; some are deep thinkers; others respond to surface attributes. Some people are engineers, and others are artists. The meta program is the way a person handles information. A second filter is a person's belief system—that person's view or theory of the world. A third filter is a person's values— his or her definition of what is right or wrong and good or bad. The forth filter is a person's memories—the events that person has lived through and experienced. The final filter is the person's past decisions. Past decisions and whether or not they worked continue to color a person's world into the future. One colleague may find your very expensive and stylish clothes to be a waste of money, whereas another may see them as a marker of someone interested in the newest and latest fashion and view that as an indicator of progressivism. Professional colleagues in midtown New York, Chicago, and Boston will most likely view you with different filters than professional colleagues in rural South Dakota or Montana. Calculate and calibrate your first impression with an eye toward the audience. There is never an opportunity to make another first impression.

Credibility

As a new practitioner, no one should expect you to perform as if you had practiced for 10 years. Trying to convey that you can function at this level is a mistake. Displaying certain attitudes and behaviors will establish your **credibility**. The first is curiosity and a willingness to learn all that is required to be effective as a clinician, an employee, and a colleague. Although no one should expect you to know everything, they will expect you to be enthused about your current circumstances. No task should be beneath you. In fact, you may be assigned such tasks as a test. Accept the requests graciously and do your best. Insisting that your credentials insulate you from some of the dirty work will poison relationships. Think of these tasks as a rite of passage. Related to this point, be cautious about insisting on being addressed by your formal title. In certain circumstances, a more formal protocol is warranted, but in private, respectful familiarity is appropriate. The second aspect of establishing credibility is to convey that you can be trusted. In this arena, actions speak louder than words. Doing what you say you will and on time is the standard. Finally, credibility is about being liked. Generally, people like to work with people who are similar to them, are familiar, have reciprocal positive feelings, and are attractive, either in appearance or personality. People like working with people who are cheerful, considerate, and generous. Research has shown that if someone is strongly disliked, competence is irrelevant because no one will work with that person. In contrast, if someone is liked coworkers will seek out every aspect of their competence (Casciaro and Lobo 2005). In other words, being liked earns you the benefit of the doubt as to competence.

Successful opening days of a career require managing the initial impression you present. Strategies for managing impressions include the following (Data from Turnley and Bolino 2001):

- **Ingratiation**: Praising others for their efforts, complimenting others, doing favors, and taking an interest in others personal lives
- **Self-promotion**: Letting others know of your talents and qualifications and how valuable you are and relating past accomplishments
- **Exemplification**: Letting others know how hard you work, taking on more than your share of work, and arriving early and staying late
- **Supplication**: Trying to gain sympathy so others will help you, acting like you know less than you do to get help, and disclosing your weaknesses
- **Intimidation**: Letting others know you will not be pushed around and dealing forcefully with others to do things your way

Using supplication and intimidation is not recommended, because one is likely to appear either needy and lazy or bossy. Handled correctly, ingratiation leads others to see you as likeable, self-promotion leads others to see you as competent, and exemplification leads others to see you as dedicated. Handle poorly, ingratiation leads others to see you as a sycophant, self-promotion leads others to see you as conceited, and exemplification leads others to see you as feeling superior.

Personal insecurity and institutional pressures to perform may entice new practitioners to behave in the way they are "supposed to" in professional situations. Such felt obligations to behave in specified ways may lead the new practitioners to try and impress others in ways that are not appropriate; the negatives of impression management detailed earlier result. Describing research you were involved with as a student establishes your credibility in an area, and boasting of its significance likely hides your insecurity. Behaving authentically is the shield from making these mistakes. You need to be self-aware enough to know your feelings and your values and astute enough to frame behaviors and impressions based on being authentic. Interacting in the workplace is akin to assuming a role; the art is to not overact. If your behavior feels fake to you, then it is, and likely appears fake to others as well.

Credibility and Mistakes

EVERYONE MAKES MISTAKES. THEY ARE inevitable. What is not inevitable is the way they are handled. First, an appropriate reaction to the mistake is required. Avoid overreacting. Acknowledge the mistake, apologize, and then get on with fixing the situation. After fixing the problem, explain what you learned and why it will not happen again. Your superiors will most likely remember not that you made a mistake, but how you fixed it.

Credibility is about integrity. One obligation of a professional is to be accountable for his or her actions. Any attempt to hide the mistake or make excuses violates one of the central elements of professional behavior, destroys credibility, and damages careers. In most of the political scandals of the recent past, it was not the behavior that got the actors in trouble, but the cover-up. In some circumstances, cover-ups may be illegal and may prompt professional board action. If you make a mistake, the impression you want to create is of a well-meaning professional who just made an error; you do not want to be viewed as an individual who lacks the integrity to "own" your mistakes.

Credibility and Not Knowing the Answer

WHEN ASKED SOMETHING YOU DO not know by a patient, the appropriate response is to be honest but convey that you have the mechanisms and willingness to provide an answer. For some clinical questions, there may be no known answer. In this case, offering a response framed by "in my best judgment" is the right response. The ethical and professional obligation for veracity is controlling in this situation.

Your response when asked something you do not know by a supervisor or a peer is different. In general, it is not a good career strategy to respond with "I don't know." Although honest, it signals lack of preparation or lack of professional competence. Having a stock response to this situation is useful. A good response to a question you do not know the answer to begins with, "Let me be sure I understand the situation." This is designed to buy some time on the assumption that the answer might come to you. Next, present what you do know about the situation and then proceed with explaining what you need to know. Follow this with what you are going to do to answer the question, and then conclude with asking when the answer is needed. The one negative statement in this sequence is sandwiched between positive statements. The positive statements will likely dominate the impression you create.

Social Media

GIVEN THE UBIQUITOUS NATURE OF the Internet and social media, caution as to what is uploaded is in order. Although you might believe that your postings are private and intended for personal audiences and acquaintances only, this may not be the case. Further, they are eternal. When applying for a supervisory position in 20 years, will the comments you make today reflect a consummate professional or a relatively immature college student whose judgment is clouded by alcohol or youthful indiscretion. Your personal presence and credibility are a function of how you look, how you talk, what you think, and how you act. But they are also a function of what you post. The Federation of State Medical Boards offers the following as guidelines for the appropriate use of social media and social networking in medical practice.

- Exercise caution in interacting with former or current patients on *personal* social networking sites.
- Only discuss clinical protocols and treatment guidelines with other practitioners on sites that have been verified to be secure and that only registered users may access.
- Patient privacy and confidentiality must be maintained at all times.
- If asked to write online about your experiences as a health professional, conflicts of interest and credentials must be revealed.

- When posting, be aware that the information may be taken out of context and further disseminated and that it remains forever.
- Use separate personal and professional networking sites.
- Report any unprofessional behavior observed online.
- The same principles of professionalism apply both online and offline.
- Cyber-bullying is inappropriate.
- Refer to your employer's policy on social networking for further clarification.

Of particular note, medical boards may levy sanctions and discipline physicians for unprofessional behavior related to social networking media.

Real Professionalism

IN HER BOOK, *CREATING PERSONAL Presence*, Dianna Booher (2011) asked how much personal presence affects credibility; for 74.5% of the respondents, the response was "a great deal." Developing presence is no mystery. According to Booher (2011), it is based on how you look, how you talk, how you think, and how you act, essentially everything about you conveys who you are.

How you look and talk are the most observable and least important. How you think and act are the least observable but most important. Although aspects of how you think and act may not be transparent, they are nevertheless observable. For the most part, you simply cannot prevent who you are as an individual, practitioner, and professional from being measured by those who interview you, hire you, work with you, and are treated by you. In other words, we all leave an intangible residue of our presence in the psyche of those we interact with. They will note us as caring or indifferent; skilled or unskilled; or reliable or erratic. Lincoln's quote is apropos: "You can fool all the people some of the time and some of the people all the time, but you cannot fool all the people all the time." That intangible personal residue emanates from our character, attitudes, and mindsets. As David Maister (2000, p. 16) observes, "Professionalism is predominantly an attitude, not a set of competencies." At a minimum, those attitudes and mindsets should include the following:

- It is not about you. In a professional context, your issues are irrelevant. It is about the patient.

- You are responsible for the outcome. There are no excuses. You must do whatever it takes.
- Civility, courtesy, and manners count. How you say and do things is important.
- There is always something more to learn. You are never a finished product.
- If you make a mistake, just fix it.
- Mankind is our business. You are there to make people's lives better. You are part of something bigger.

The impression we want to manage, create, and leave with our audiences is not so much someone with the outer manifestations of a professional, but someone with the heart of a professional. It will show through.

Conclusion

THIS CHAPTER ASKS YOU TO consider how you present yourself, the image you create, and whether that image is a professional one. It conveys that the essence of establishing credibility is enthusiasm and integrity. Specific recommendations on dealing with social media, mistakes, and lack of knowledge are offered.

What Do the Practitioners/Others Say?

FOR NEXT CLASS, BE PREPARED to discuss creating impressions based on any *one* of the following:

- A discussion with your colleagues, or others, on how they feel and what they know about establishing credibility.
- An article on personal presence or impression management, either from the research literature or any other source.
- A movie, television program, or YouTube video about establishing credibility or first impressions.
- A book on personal presence (literary, historical, psychological, or any other source).

Personal Learning Plan: Impressions

USE THE FOLLOWING GUIDE TO develop a personal learning plan for yourself on establishing credibility.

What prompted you to develop this plan?	
What is the general area for improvement?	
What is the specific issue for improvement?	
Why is this important to you?	
How do you generally act in these areas?	
What are your goals?	
What strategies are required?	
Who/what is necessary to meet your goals with this strategy?	
How will you measure success/failure with this effort?	
How will you reflect and capture the lesson from this effort that can be generalized to other circumstances?	

The Students: Personal and Professional Issues

B ASED ON THE DESCRIPTION OF each student at the beginning of the chapter, what are the personal and professional issues (either immediately or in the future) confronting each student? Consider whether they are linked and, if so, how. Finally, what would you recommend to each student to resolve these issues?

Dana S.

Personal Issues

Professional Issues

Are They Linked? Will the Personal Issues Impact Professional Behavior?

Recommendations

Ivan T.

Personal Issues

Professional Issues

Are They Linked? Will the Personal Issues Impact Professional Behavior?

Recommendations

Niki M.

Personal Issues

Professional Issues

Are They Linked? Will the Personal Issues Impact Professional Behavior?

Recommendations

Ryan P.

Personal Issues

Professional Issues

Are They Linked? Will the Personal Issues Impact Professional Behavior?

Recommendations

Exercises

1. With several of your classmates develop guidelines for the following:

   Acceptable dress in school; in a professional setting.

   Acceptable grooming in school; in a professional setting.

   Acceptable punctuality in school; in a professional setting.

   Acceptable social media behaviors in school; in a professional setting.

   Acceptable verbal interactions (humor, etc.) in school; in a professional setting.

   Acceptable etiquette in school; in a professional setting.

   Acceptable written communications in school; in a professional setting.

   Acceptable cell phone etiquette in school; in a professional setting.

2. Develop a mechanism to share these guidelines with one another.

3. Write a one-page executive summary of the chapter.

4. Review the mind map from the opening of the chapter. Would you change anything following reading the chapter?

What's Important to You in the Chapter?

WITH SEVERAL OF YOUR CLASSMATES, discuss the idea or ideas most likely to effect a change in your values, attitudes, or behaviors. Be succinct. Write no more than two sentences.

References

Booher, D. (2011). *Creating Personal Presence*. San Francisco, CA: Berret-Koehler.

Casciaro, T., and Lobo, M. S. (2005). Competent jerks, lovable fools, and the formation of social networks. *Harvard Business Review*. June, 1–8.

Maister, D. H. (2000). *True Professionalism*. New York: Touchstone.

Turnley, W. H., and Bolino, M. C. (2001). Achieving desired images while avoiding undesired images: Exploring the role of self-monitoring in impression management. *Journal of Applied Psychology.* 86 (2), 351–360.

Suggested Readings

Bixler, S., and Scherrer Dugan, L. (2001). *5 Steps to Professional Presence.* Avon, MA: Adams Media Corp.

Boothman, N. (2008). *How to Make People Like You in 90 Seconds.* New York: Workman Publishing.

Kasar, J., and Nelson Clark, E. (2000). *Developing Professional Behaviors.* Thorofare, NJ: SLACK Inc.

Key, J. R. (2012). *Journey Towards Professionalism.* Bloomington, IN: iUniverse.

Monarth, H. (2012). *Executive Presence.* New York: McGraw-Hill.

Sanders, T. (2006). *The Likeability Factor.* New York: Three Rivers Press.

Templar, R. (2005). *The Rules of Work.* Upper Saddle River, NJ: FT Press.

Wiersma, B. (2011). *The Power of Professionalism.* Los Altos, CA: Ravel Media.

CHAPTER 10

Professionalism as a Student

Preassessment: Professionalism as a Student

Mind Mapping

*Consider the term displayed on the page. For this term, without thinking or editing, write down the ideas, concepts, examples, contradictions, and theories that come to mind. Do not arrange them in any systematic or orderly manner. Scatter them about the page. Now, draw lines between your additions indicating that there is a relationship between the terms. If something causes something else, indicate this with an arrow. Relationships may be reciprocal, meaning both cause each other, requiring arrows at both ends. Indicate the strength of the relationships by darkening and thickening the lines; stronger relationships have darker and thicker lines. **Most important: There is no right answer. Do not compare with your classmates.** What you have is a mind map, your mental representation of these topics. Review to determine if anything has changed following this section.*

Student Obligations

The Students

I

D ANA S. HAD NEVER BEEN so angry. The course she was taking now was exceedingly difficult for her. She spent hours and hours studying and preparing only to barely pass the examination. Whether she could pass the course hinged on two or three questions on each exam. Currently, her score for the course was 71.3%, with a score of 69.5% required to pass. The stress was relentless. She couldn't let up for a single lecture or study session. It frightened Dana to think that her career and her life could come down to only three or four questions over a semester.

Word had begun to circulate about one of her classmates. The informal student grapevine buzzed with the brazenness of the cheating of one of the students. This was more than a quick glance at another student's test or an overly collaborative lab effort. This student was sneaking his cell phone out during the test and accessing the complete set of notes for the course. At first, Dana didn't believe it. How could anyone be so brazen and not get caught? The tests were monitored by graduate assistants who would often be distracted talking to one another or reviewing their own work. Dana decided to sit behind this student during one of the exams. During the exam, she saw him pull his phone out and scroll through notes before answering some of the questions. Dana also knew this student had a spotty record of class attendance. Dana reflected on how all her hours of preparation could be negated by a few snapshots of the class notes. The word was that this student had been scoring in the high 80s on the exams. He never seemed stressed.

Outside of class after the last exam, several students had congregated and were discussing approaching the administration about this problem. They asked Dana if she wanted to join them. This would be no anonymous note to the administration, but a face-to-face meeting. Dana was torn.

II

Even though Ivan T. was on clinical rotations, he was also working weekend hours at a health facility. Last night, the frustration of his busy schedule got to him. It had been a long week. He was still dealing with his father's death, he began to suspect that his girlfriend wanted to end their relationship, and he just got his bill for next semester's tuition. In addition to all this, he had a bad case of the flu but couldn't afford to take off work.

As he was checking in for work, the supervisor asked why he was 5 minutes late. Ivan lost his composure, punched the time clock off the wall, and stormed out of the facility. It was now 8 hours later, and the import of what he had done began to sink in. He was extremely embarrassed. This was not the first Ivan had lost his temper. However, all the other incidents had been at home or occurred in his private life.

Ivan began to ponder what to do, who to talk to, and what to say. Ivan sensed this was a pivotal moment in his career. He was worried he would be fired for this incident. He also hated feeling so tense all the time.

III

Niki M. had always been at the top academically. She had earned all A's in high school, only one B as an undergraduate, and only two B's in the professional program. Niki looked at her final grade for the course—a B, not even a B+. Niki was meeting with the instructor with her tests in hand. She asked the instructor to reread all of her answers. The instructor glanced at the tests and said, "I remember your exams explicitly. You simply did not understand three or four critical points. There is no reason for me to reread them. In fact, I think I was fairly generous with my grade."

The instructor simply could not be swayed to alter Niki's grade or reread her tests. After about 15 minutes of back-and-forth sparring, the instructor declared, "Look I'm not going to change the grade just because you have always had A's. I have your scores recorded, and they will stand. I think the meeting is over." Niki tried to continue the meeting. Finally, the exasperated instructor said, "You have the right to be heard. You don't have the right to have everything you want. You've been heard. I have a family to like me; I don't need you to like me. This meeting is over." With that, the instructor got up from her desk, took Niki's coat off the hook, handed it to her, and opened the door. Niki walked past her and said, "For the money I spent on this course, I should have a better grade, and certainly I should have better instruction from you. You should hear what the students say about you as a teacher and the way you dress." She slammed the door and walked out.

IV

Even though he knew it would ultimately benefit his family to return to school, Ryan P. felt guilty about the time it took away from his family, especially his daughters. Although Ryan had always been organized, his time was so constrained now that he found he had to become super organized. At the beginning of the semester, Ryan reviewed test dates and assignments and allocated the amount of time required for each. He also allocated time for all family events that would happen during the semester. He was so detailed that he had allocated 3 hours to shop for the food for Thanksgiving dinner.

During class that day, Ryan couldn't believe his ears. The junior faculty member just announced he thought it would be a good exercise for the class to write a five-page paper over the weekend on the topic they had been discussing. This assignment was in addition to those he had been assigned at the beginning of the semester. The instructor commented that the assignment shouldn't take more than 3 or 4 hours. The class went into an uproar at the announcement. Ryan found himself taking on the role as spokesman for the class. At first, his comments were appropriate and respectful. But as he talked, he remembered that he told his daughter he would be at her soccer game this weekend. This assignment would mean he would have to miss it. Ryan sensed he was about to lose his composure and "go off" on the instructor.

🔹 LEARNING OBJECTIVES

- Describe attitudes that conflict with professionalism as a student.
- Discuss emotional intelligence and student professionalism.
- Discuss cognitive restructuring and student professionalism.

🔹 KEY TERMS

- Academic dishonesty
- Academic entitlement
- Academic incivility

- Psychological contract
- Student consumerism

Professional or Student?

MOST PEOPLE READING THIS BOOK think of themselves as professional students. The phrase *professional student* has two connotations: an individual who prolongs education to avoid having to go to work, and an individual pursuing a professional degree. The second connotation is the focus here. Often, there is a tendency to emphasize the *student* aspect of the phrase rather than the *professional* aspect because the role of a student is familiar and the concerns are immediate. However, whether students realize it or not, their voluntary matriculation into a program obligates them to the same professional standards as graduate, licensed practitioners. *This is not a matter of choice.* Although students may be initiates and novices, they are professionals nevertheless and have professional obligations and standards that extend to the classroom, the laboratory, the experiential site, relationships with faculty, staff, and administrators, and any other academic pursuits.

Factors That Diminish Professionalism

STUDENT CONSUMERISM IS THE VIEW, held by students and others, that college is just another consumer marketplace and a university education is just another product. This view is characterized by students' comments such as, "I am paying for this course, so I am paying your salary" or "It is your job to teach and make sure I get the grade I want." If the student is displeased, uncomfortable, or bored, it is the instructor's fault. Students approach university education with certain expectations and aspirations. Students may seek cultural capital (knowledge learned in the classroom), social capital (the personal networks acquired in college that may be instrumental in their careers), and economic capital (the financial benefits to be gained from college and the degree obtained).

The various perspectives may influence expectations and behaviors. The idea of college as another consumer marketplace may be driven by the significant financial investment students and families make.

Academic Entitlement

ACADEMIC ENTITLEMENT IS THE IDEA that one deserves a grade or special treatment regardless of his or her input and performance. Academic entitlement includes the belief that (1) knowledge is a right and the student should receive it with minimal exertion or discomfort, (2) the instructor will provide all the necessary requirements for success, (3) the instructor is responsible for student success or failure, (4) students should receive recognition regardless of the effort expended, and (5) confrontations with instructors and administrators is acceptable if expectations are not met. Academic entitlement may result due to unearned praise from parents and teachers when young. The relative grade inflation of the last generation may reinforce the notion that grades are given rather than earned. Academic entitlement may be a self-serving coping strategy when students are unable to meet the rigor of college-level courses. Further, personality may be related to a sense of academic entitlement. Specifically, students low in agreeableness and conscientiousness may exhibit a sense of entitlement. Students with an unrealistic and grandiose assessment of their abilities and narcissists may have tendencies toward entitlement. Students with a high sense of entitlement believe that responsibility for their performance resides outside themselves and that they do not have either the ability or the obligation to perform.

Academic Incivility

ANY ACTIVITY THAT DISRUPTS THE learning environment of the classroom, distracts other students or the instructor, or is rude may be viewed as **academic incivility**. Generally, these activities include behaviors such as overt disengagement, generally disruptive acts, or specific acts directed at the instructor. Academic incivility may also include overt and egregious subversions of the learning process such as alcohol or illicit drug use, plagiarism, or cheating. Specific incivilities include such things as being late, talking in class, eating in class, sleeping in class, inattention, using cell phones, in general any activity that compromises the student or the instructor in the pursuit of learning. (Nilson and Jackson 2004):

Academic incivility by students may be due to a general deterioration in civility in society at large, overly permissive parents, the need for instant gratification, insufficient rigor and discipline at the high school level, illness, fatigue, stress, emotional immaturity, medication or substance abuse, personal problems, misplaced aggression, increased class sizes, inexperienced or adjunct faculty, specific instructor attributes (e.g., age, gender, ethnicity, status within the university), incivility on the part of faculty, faculty incompetence, overly sensitive faculty, and modern communication technology (Knepp 2012).

Academic Dishonesty

A N EXTREME FORM OF ACADEMIC incivility is **academic dishonesty**. Academic dishonesty is not only unprofessional, but also unethical. Academic dishonesty is taking a "cognitive shortcut" by submitting work for assessment that is not your own. It is misconduct to gain an advantage. The reasons students give for cheating may be ignorance of the topic, poor professors and teaching environment, inadequate policies and penalties for cheating, the desire for a better grade, opportunity, technology that makes it easier, procrastination, underdeveloped moral reasoning, desire for a good job, and a culture that encourages cheating (Wideman 2011). Academic dishonesty is viewed as having gradations of seriousness. Copying someone's homework assignment is different from buying a written PhD dissertation. An extension of the academic dishonesty debate is the dilemma of knowing and reporting classmates who are cheating. Depending on the type of academic dishonesty considered, the rate of dishonesty varies from approximately 15% to over 65% of all students. Some might argue that academic dishonesty is a "victimless" crime. However, there is evidence to suggest that academic dishonesty today foreshadows unethical, unprofessional, and illegal activities later in practice (Laduke 2012).

Case for Professionalism in School

M OST STUDENTS FIND THEMSELVES IN a complex web of relationships and obligations. Some students may be relatively young with minimal responsibilities, whereas others may be well along in life with significant career and family obligations as they advance their careers through additional training and education. Whatever the circumstances, in terms of professional growth, the student is obligated to apply the same standards for professionalism to the academic context as they would later to the work context. In one view, school can be viewed as the "job" for the novice professional. School is the professional practice site. School is where the professional obligations for altruism, accountability, duty, honor, integrity, excellence, and respect for others are not only learned, but also first applied and practiced. School can be viewed as a laboratory where the standards for these traits are experimented with and inculcated into personal attitudes, values, and behaviors. Excellence and accountability to a high school student are completely different from excellence and accountability to a perfusionist, nurse, or pharmacist, where the penalty for failure may be catastrophic. Professionalism is a habit and needs to be practiced. It does not begin at graduation. The penalty for lack of professionalism after graduation may be dismissal from a job; the penalty in school may be relatively minor, such as bruised emotions, ruffled relationships, and diminished assessments. In other words, school is a place to practice professionalism and what it means, where the consequences of getting it wrong are minimal. Acting professionally as a student is not a matter of choice—it is an ethical obligation of a novice in the profession.

Student Professionalism as a Career Strategy

SIX MONTHS AFTER YOU START your job, those you work with and for will have sized you up. The comments may be something such as, "This person is going to be a good fit; she is great with the patients, she knows their stuff, and everyone likes to work with her," or "This person is good with the patients and really knows his stuff, but he is hard to work with." This informal assessment influences how people see your progression in the profession. One could be marked for advancement and greater responsibility, slotted as an effective practitioner only, or seen as someone who is likely to have trouble in his or her career. In fact, this "reading" of a person begins in school. Faculty, advisors, and preceptors are an interconnected network of contacts, friends, and references that are likely to travel in the same circles and attend the same conferences and meetings. It is foolish to prejudice that assessment by careless and unprofessional behavior as a student. A poor result on a test followed by a willingness to accept responsibility, rather than blame out; attentive engagement in the classroom; and civility in dealing with staff create impressions that are remembered. Generally, it is the extremes of student behavior that get noted. If you are remembered as a student who is a problem, then the behavior is usually egregious. Although faculty and advisors want to see you do well, they cannot change the truth about you or lie on your behalf. If asked directly about you, they will simply not say anything at all if their impression is less than favorable. Such approaches are easily read for what they are. Conversely, most faculty will be effusive in their praise of you if it is warranted. You are going to make enemies in life and work and disappoint people inadvertently; it makes no sense to do it knowingly. As one district manager advised student interns when they were hired, you are now on a 4-year job interview. This does not mean you have to get it right every day in every interaction, but acknowledging missteps and acting accordingly are the marks of a professional.

Personal Growth in School

THERE IS NO QUESTION THAT school is a stressful experience. The constant assessment, scrutiny, and demand on time are wearing. Often money and family issues add to the struggle. Meanwhile, life goes on. Each student has worked out more or less functional behavioral patterns for dealing with stress, fear, worry, test anxiety, perfectionism, public speaking, various work and personal relationships, how they think, how they get things done, making decisions, procrastination, values, emotions, and so on. F. Scott Fitzgerald observed that, "The test of a first rate intelligence is the ability to hold two opposing ideas in the mind at the same time and still retain the ability to function." The two opposing ideas are these: as you are today is just fine, but if you want to grow, you need to change.

School is a valuable laboratory for conscious personal growth with the possibility for experimentation and where the consequences for failure are relatively minor. Although a botched presentation feels catastrophic at the time, in reality, it is insignificant over a lifetime. The astute student uses school not just to become technically proficient, but to experiment with new patterns of thought and behavior. Personal growth as a student requires leaning into the discomfort of new patterns of thought and behavior related to yourself. Once shy does not mandate always shy. Practicing new patterns of thought and behavior in the benign atmosphere of school is preferable to developing new patterns of thought and behavior in the rough and tumble of practice. If an instructor challenges you, pushes you, or makes you uncomfortable, whether deserved or not, it is not a cause for anger, but a prod to growth. Attention from an instructor is an indication of the instructor's belief in your potential. View it as such. A central premise of this book is that you cannot separate the clinician/practitioner from the individual. Use school to stretch yourself, challenge yourself, and develop yourself—it is your professional obligation.

Student Professionalism and Emotional Intelligence

CONSIDER A RETURNED EXAM THAT you just barely failed due to what you believe to be unfair test questions and questionable grading. The worst possible way to handle this situation would be to burst into the instructor's office angry and accusatory, go see the dean of students, and call your parents and ask them to call the dean of the school. Now, view this situation from an emotional intelligence framework. Emotional intelligence is about understanding your emotions and those of another person and then crafting a behavior appropriate to the context. Emotionally intelligent individuals first understand themselves. A failed exam is traumatic; take some time, a day or more, to compose your thoughts and work through your emotions. Emotionally intelligent people also take time to understand the other person. They take time to think how the instructor will react if they confront them, go over the instructor's head, or bring their parents into the picture. It is unlikely the instructor's feelings about this approach will be favorable to their case. They imagine how they would feel if they were in the instructor's shoes. They read the context and situation. They find a time in the week when the instructor is not pressured by something else and when the instructor will have time for this issue and likely to be in a good mood. Emotionally intelligent students understand the parameters of what is acceptable in a relationship between instructor and student.

Now, consider how to approach the instructor. What should your demeanor be? How do you get the instructor on your side? What do you say? Emotionally intelligent students acknowledge their ultimate responsibility for the outcome. They frame the conversation as wanting to understand and to get better, rather than "lawyering up" for a few points. They never threaten and never pressure. They understand that although this conversation is over a few points, it is also the beginning of what might be a productive professional relationship if the interaction is handled correctly. *Emotionally intelligent* people craft behaviors that get them what they want and let them win. *Emotionally unintelligent* people act out and lose.

Psychological Contracts

A PSYCHOLOGICAL CONTRACT IS A PERSON'S beliefs about the terms of an exchange between two parties. In this context, it is the student's beliefs (expectations) about what the educational process is about. Many of those beliefs are appropriate. It is appropriate to expect and anticipate that good work will be rewarded, that you will be treated fairly and with an appropriate level of civility, and that the educational process will prepare you for practice. When this contract is violated, it is appropriate to be upset, disappointed, and even angry. It is something else to believe you have a right to certain grades and to never be inconvenienced or challenged, to believe that you deserve these things, and to be entitled. To be upset, disappointed, or angry at these circumstances is not appropriate. Practice, and life itself, will have its disappointments; the expectations of a 20-year-old give way to an understanding of what practice and life is about. Many aspects of life and practice will be unfair. Accepting this inevitability is a mark of maturity and wisdom; it is the path to making a first-rate clinician, and that path begins in school.

Conclusion

THIS CHAPTER ASKS STUDENTS TO consider themselves as professionals, with the attendant obligations of the profession. Academic entitlement is discussed along with academic incivility and academic dishonesty.

The case is made for professionalism in school and student professionalism as a career strategy. Personal growth, student professionalism and emotional intelligence, and psychological contracts are also discussed.

What Do the Practitioners/Others Say?

FOR NEXT CLASS, BE PREPARED to discuss professionalism as a student based on any *one* of the following:

- A discussion with your colleagues, or others, on how they feel and what they know about professionalism as a student.
- An article on student professionalism, either from the research literature or any other source.
- A movie, television program, or YouTube video about student professionalism.
- A book on student professionalism (literary, historical, psychological, or any other source).

Personal Learning Plan: Student Professionalism

Use the following guide to develop a personal learning plan for yourself on establishing credibility.

What prompted you to develop this plan?	
What is the general area for improvement?	
What is the specific issue for improvement?	
Why is this important to you?	
How do you generally act in these areas?	
What are your goals?	
What strategies are required?	
Who/what is necessary to meet your goals with this strategy?	
How will you measure success/failure with this effort?	
How will you reflect and capture the lesson from this effort that can be generalized to other circumstances?	

The Students: Personal and Professional Issues

BASED ON THE DESCRIPTION OF each student at the beginning of the chapter, what are the personal and professional issues (either immediately or in the future) confronting each student? Consider if they are linked and, if so, how. Finally, what would you recommend to each student to resolve these issues?

Dana S.

Personal Issues

Professional Issues

Are They Linked? Will the Personal Issues Impact Professional Behavior?

Recommendations

Ivan T.

Personal Issues

Professional Issues

Are They Linked? Will the Personal Issues Impact Professional Behavior?

Recommendations

Niki M.

Personal Issues

Professional Issues

Are They Linked? Will the Personal Issues Impact Professional Behavior?

Recommendations

Ryan P.

Personal Issues

Professional Issues

Are They Linked? Will the Personal Issues Impact Professional Behavior?

Recommendations

Exercises

Academic Entitlement

Please consider whether you agree or disagree with the following statements.

It is unnecessary for me to participate in class when the professor is paid for teaching, not for asking questions.

If I miss class, it is my responsibility to get the notes.

I am not motivated to put a lot of effort into group work because another member will end up doing it.

I believe that the university does not provide me with the resources I need to succeed in college.

Most professors do not really know what they are talking about.

If I do poorly in a course and I could not make my professor's office hours, the fault lies with the professor.

I believe that it is my responsibility to seek out the resources to succeed in college.

For group assignments, it is acceptable to take a back seat and let others do most of the work if I am busy.

For group work, I should receive the same grade as the other group members regardless of my level of effort.

Professors are employees who just get money for teaching.

My professors are obligated to help me prepare for exams.

Professors must be entertaining to be good.

My professors should reconsider my grade if I am close to the grade I want.

I should never receive a zero on an assignment that I turned in.

My professors should curve my grade if I am close to the next letter grade.

Psychological Entitlement

Please consider whether you agree or disagree with the following statements about yourself.

1. I honestly feel I'm just more deserving than others.
2. Great things should come to me.
3. If I were on the *Titanic*, I would deserve to be on the first lifeboat.
4. I demand the best because I am worth it.
5. I do not necessarily deserve special treatment.
6. I deserve more things in my life.
7. People like me deserve an extra break now and then.
8. Things should go my way.
9. I feel entitled to more of everything.

Campbell, W. K., Bonacci, A. M., Shelton, J., Exline, J. J., and Bushman, B. J. (2004). Psychological entitlement: Interpersonal consequences and validation of a self-report measure. *Journal of Personality Assessment.* 83 (1), 29–45.

Discussion Questions

1. Do you believe cheating in school foreshadows cheating in practice?
2. Under what circumstances is it permissible to leave a class early? How should it be handled?
3. If you believe an instructor is rude to you, how should you handle it?
4. Are there circumstances where it is reasonable to look at your phone during a lecture?
5. How would you feel if your instructor looked at their phone during your presentation?
6. Are there circumstances where it is permissible to eat in class? How should it be handled?
7. Are there circumstances where it is acceptable to go over an instructor's head?

8. You have consistently been at the top of your class academically, but the instructor refuses to write a letter of recommendation due to what she terms your unprofessionalism. What do you do?

9. Are there ever circumstances where you should apologize to an instructor?

10. What would you do if there is rampant cheating in a classroom. Would your response change if the grades were curved rather than graded on a scale? If the cheater was a friend? If you knew your friend needed to pass the course to graduate?

11. When is it okay to ask an instructor to grade you up?

12. Should you ever consider the professor's feelings in dealing with him or her?

13. Is it okay to attack a professor on a course evaluation?

14. If you had problems with an instructor, would you ask your parents to intervene?

15. Imagine you are in a boring class with an inept instructor that is scheduled right before another class in which you are taking a mid-term exam. Imagine your feelings of boredom, anxiety, anger, and tension. Consider the worst possible way for you to handle this situation, such as acting out in class, leaving in a huff, or pulling out your notes for the next class. Consider how to handle this situation from an emotional intelligence perspective. Consider how to handle this situation using cognitive reappraisal.

16. If the faculty were sitting at lunch and your name came up, what do you think they would say about you? Would they even know who you are?

17. Write a one-paragraph character sketch of five members of your faculty. How is this useful if you had an issue with one of them?

Cheating Behaviors

Please answer yes if you think the following behaviors are OK or no if not to the following statements.

1. Paraphrasing material from another source without acknowledging the original author. _____

2. Inventing data (i.e., entering nonexistent results into the database). _____

3. Allowing own coursework to be copied by another student. _____

4. Fabricating references or a bibliography. _____

5. Copying material for coursework from a book or other publication without acknowledging the source. _____

6. Altering data (e.g., adjusting data to obtain a significant result). _____

7. Copying another student's coursework with the student's knowledge. _____

8. Ensuring the availability of books or journal articles in the library by deliberately misshelving them so other students cannot find them or by cutting out the relevant article or chapter. _____

9. In a situation where students mark each other's work, coming to an agreement with another student or students to mark each other's work more generously than it merits. _____

10. Submitting a piece of coursework as an individual piece of work when it has actually been written jointly with another student. _____

11. Doing another student's coursework for them. _____

12. Copying from a neighbor during an examination without them realizing. _____

13. Lying about medical or other circumstances to get an extended deadline or exemption from a piece of work. _____

14. Taking unauthorized material into an examination (e.g., cribs). _____

15. Illicitly gaining advance information about the contents of an examination paper. _____

16. Copying another student's coursework without the student's knowledge. _____

17. Submitting coursework from an outside source (e.g., a former student offers to sell pre-prepared essays; "essay banks'). _____

18. Premeditated collusion between two or more students to communicate answers to each other during an examination. _____

19. Lying about medical or other circumstances to get special consideration by examiners (e.g., getting the exam board to take a more lenient view of results; extra time to complete the exam). _____

20. Attempting to obtain special consideration by offering or receiving favors through, for example, bribery, seduction, or corruption. _____

21. Taking an examination for someone else or having someone else take an examination for you. _____

Calculate your cheating index as the percentage of yes answers to total questions (21). What does this percentage say about you? Are there implications in this for future practice? Do you consider any of the above items not to be cheating?

Newstead, S. E., Franklyn-Stokes, A., and Armstead, P. (1996). Individual differences in student cheating. *Journal of Educational Psychology*. 88 (2), 232.

1. Imagine the final paper in your final class is due in a few days and you have not started. Would it be acceptable to buy a paper if the reason for not having the paper is:

   Procrastination

   Worked too much

   Personal or family illness

   Do not want to write paper

   Used the weekend before for personal holiday

2. Write a one-page executive summary of the chapter.

3. Review the mind map from the opening of the chapter. Would you change anything after reading the chapter?

What's Important to You in the Chapter?

WITH SEVERAL OF YOUR CLASSMATES, discuss the idea or ideas that are most likely to effect a change in your values, attitudes, or behaviors. Be succinct. Write no more than two sentences. If Blackboard is used in your class, post your important ideas to the site.

References

Campbell, W. K., Bonacci, A. M., Shelton, J., Exline, J. J., and Bushman, B. J. (2004). Psychological entitlement: Interpersonal consequences and validation of a self-report measure. *Journal of Personality Assessment*. 83 (1), 29–45.

Knepp, K. A. F. (2012). Understanding student and faculty incivility in higher education. *The Journal of Effective Teaching*. 12 (1), 32–45.

Laduke, R. D. (2012). Academic dishonesty today, unethical practices tomorrow? *Journal of Professional Nursing*. 29 (6), 402–406.

Nilson, L. B., and Jackson, N. S. (June, 2004). Combating classroom misconduct (incivility) with bills of rights. Paper presented at the International Consortium for Educational Development, Ottawa, Ontario, Canada.

Wideman, M. (2011). Caring or collusion? Academic dishonesty in a school of nursing. *Canadian Journal of Higher Education*. 41 (2), 28–43.

Suggested Readings

Berger, B. A., ed. (2003). *Promoting Civility in Pharmacy Education*. Binghamton, NY: Pharmaceutical Products Press.

Boswell, S. S. (2012). "I *deserve* success": Academic entitlement attitudes and their relationships with course self-efficacy, social networking, and demographic variables. *Social Psychology in Education*. 15, 353–365.

Cain, J., Romanelli, F., and Smith, K. M. (2012). Academic entitlement in pharmacy education. *American Journal of Pharmaceutical Education*. 76 (10), 1–8.

Chowning, K., and Campbell, N. J. (2009). Development and validation of a measure of academic entitlement: Individual differences in student's externalized responsibility and entitled expectations. *Journal of Educational Psychology*. 101 (4), 982–997.

Ciani, K. D., Summers, J. J., and Easter, M. A. (2008). Gender differences in academic entitlement among college students. *The Journal of Genetic Psychology*. 169 (4), 332–344.

Clark, C. M., and Springer, P. J. (2007). Thoughts on incivility: Student and faculty perceptions of uncivil behavior in nursing education. *Nursing Education Perspective*. 28 (2), 93–97.

Delucchi, M., and Korgen, K. (2002). "We're the customers—We pay the tuition": Student consumerism among undergraduate sociology majors. *Teaching Sociology*. 30, 100–107.

Greenberger, E., Lessard, J., Chen, C., and Farruggia, S. P. (2008). Self-entitled students: Contributions of personality, parenting, and motivational factors. *Journal of Youth and Adolescence*. 37, 1193–1204.

Mellor, J. K. (2011). Academic entitlement and incivility: Differences in faculty and student perceptions. Unpublished dissertation. University of Arizona.

Saunders, D. B. (2014). Exploring a customer orientation: Free-market logic and college students. *The Review of Higher Education.* 37 (2), 197–219.

Sutton, G., and Griffin, M. A. (2004). Integrating expectations, experiences, and psychological contract violations: A longitudinal study of new professionals. *Journal of Occupational and Organizational Psychology.* 77, 493–514.

Taylor, C., Farver, C., and Stoller, J. K. (2011). Can emotional intelligence training serve as an alternative approach to teaching professionalism to residents? *Academic Medicine.* 86 (12), 1551–1554.

CHAPTER
11

Professionalism
at Work

Preassessment: Professionalism at Work

Mind Mapping

Consider the term displayed on the page. For this term, without thinking or editing, write down the ideas, concepts, examples, contradictions, and theories that come to mind. Do not arrange them in any systematic or orderly manner. Scatter them about the page. Now, draw lines between your additions indicating that there is a relationship between the terms. If something causes something else, indicate this with an arrow. Relationships may be reciprocal, meaning both cause each other, requiring arrows at both ends. Indicate the strength of the relationships by darkening and thickening the lines; stronger relationships have darker and thicker lines. **Most important: There is no right answer. Do not compare with your classmates.** *What you have is a mind map, your mental representation of these topics. Review to determine if anything has changed following this section.*

Work

The Students

I

As she had hoped, dana S. found a job upon graduation in a small healthcare facility only 40 miles from her mother's home. It was perfect; it was close enough to see her mother when she wanted, but not so close that her mother could easily drop in. Through a small inheritance from her grandmother, Dana had enough money for a down payment on a small house. It was also perfect, a 1940s cottage. Much of the renovation had already been completed, but several rooms still needed upgrading, including the kitchen. Despite the 40 miles, Dana's mother had taken to driving by and bombarding her with pictures and ideas for the renovations. So far, Dana had been able to handle her mother's involvement, but she sensed that a major conflict was brewing. She appreciated her mother's help and, in fact, needed some of it, but she wanted to have the final word on the decisions.

Because she worked at a small facility, Dana was pushed to assume as much responsibility at work as possible. She had been tasked with supervising the night shift. There were four technicians on this shift, who were all older and more experienced than Dana. Last night when Dana asked one of the technicians to do something, the technician told her, "No. I don't feel like doing it. I know what needs to be done, and you are not qualified to be supervising me." Dana didn't know what to say to the technician.

II

All his life, Ivan T. had never had any extra money. He blamed his father for that. His family had always just barely gotten by. When a company held out a signing bonus, Ivan jumped at it. He couldn't imagine having that much money, and now it was in his bank account. He spent many pleasant hours anticipating how he would spend it. He only spent a small amount to buy some new clothes for work. He knew he wanted to make a good first impression.

The first weeks at work were eye opening. During the interviews, the recruiter had regaled him with the numerous clinical activities that he could become involved in and the initiatives that were under way. Ivan wondered if he had actually heard those things. He seemed to be working in a parallel universe. Ivan noticed that a lot of the staff who had been at the company for a long time seemed angry. The rest of the staff seemed to come and go. One day at the end of his shift, he asked one of the long-time workers who was close to retirement about the situation. His coworker replied, "I'm not usually this direct, but I will be gone in 2 months, so this is the story. This place is about money, pure and simple. Churn and earn. It wasn't that way when I started, and I think it's only going to get worse. But, if you can stick it out, you can make good money."

Soon after taking the job, the regimentation of the job started to bother Ivan. He remembered the incident with the time clock. Ivan began to think he may not be a good fit for this job. He thought about calling his old professor, the one who had suggested he should go on to school. Ivan sensed he needed to make a decision.

III

It felt good to have graduated. Niki M. had managed to put herself through school, land a job in a major metropolitan area, and raise her son. Her parents had been helpful and were there in an emergency if she needed them, but they were not indulgent. Their attitude had always been that people have to live with their choices. Counting her undergraduate degree, Niki had been in school for 8 years. Recently, she had met some classmates from high school, women who she thought were much less accomplished than her. One classmate had gone to beautician school for 1 year and was now making over $80,000 per year cutting hair. She was a wonderful person, warm and caring. Niki understood why her salary was at that level and planned to have her former classmate start cutting her hair. Niki would just make that salary in her first year out of school, and she had loans to repay. In addition, when she approached her ex-husband about establishing a college fund for their son, he was less than cooperative.

Niki began to feel that it was now her turn to indulge herself. She replaced her old car and finally began to upgrade her wardrobe. She would live 1 or 2 months more in her parents' basement and then start to look for a new place to live. She hadn't really noticed him when he got on the elevator. They both listened to the comments of two student interns discussing their social lives. As they approached the last floor, and the students got off, it was only the two of them. In a quiet voice, he asked if she was amused or bemused by the students. She noticed him now. As he got off the elevator, Niki knew she wanted to find out more about him.

IV

Ryan P. was reflecting on how he got to this stage of his life. He had 1 year to go to finish the program. He was confident now that he would make it. He remembered how he had gotten into his former profession, the telecommunications industry. It was a summer job doing manual labor. He made $10.00 per hour. That was good money when he was in college. Because he was a hard worker and conscientious, he was offered a full-time job when he graduated. It was so easy. He didn't have to interview, move away from home, or go through any of the normal rites of passage that graduating college students go through. With the new job, he felt secure. He asked his high school sweetheart to marry him. Within 2 years of graduation, Ryan had a house, a wife, and a baby on the way. The only problem, Ryan recalled, was that he began to feel like he had sold himself short. Maybe he could have been more, but with the family responsibilities, Ryan had no choice but to continue with this path.

School had been a struggle, but Ryan had never felt better about himself. Although his bank accounts were depleted, his sense of accomplishment and satisfaction with himself had never been higher. As his oldest child was about to graduate from college and his youngest child about to enter college, Ryan wanted to give them advice about their careers based on his experience. His conclusion, though it seemed simple, was this—the secret to work and careers is to just do what you want.

⁘ LEARNING OBJECTIVES

- Describe the assumptions in managing your boss.
- Discuss how to shape your boss's behavior.
- Describe what supervisors do.
- Describe mistakes that supervisors tend to make.
- Discuss the facts of organizational life.
- Discuss emotional intelligence and politics.
- Discuss gossip at work.
- Describe how to recognize a toxic work environment.

- Discuss the issues related to romantic relationships at work.
- Discuss culture at work.

✦ KEY TERMS

- Culture
- Prudent paranoia
- Toxic political environment

Work

HEALTH CARE IS A PROFESSION and a moral enterprise; it is also a job. A generation ago, many healthcare practitioners worked in relatively small organizations or with sole practitioners. That has largely changed. Much of health care today is corporate. Many healthcare practitioners are employees rather than entrepreneurs. Many are shift workers. Work is an exchange. You are there to add economic value in excess of the cost of your salary. You are neither entitled nor guaranteed a job. Job security emanates, for everyone in the healthcare system—chief executive officer (CEO) to housekeeping—from satisfying the wants and demands of the consumer. In exchange for this, you should get what you want from the organization. Your aspirations may be to move to the upper echelons of the organization or work part time to raise your family. Do not feel guilty. This is your part of the exchange.

Generally, the demands of professionalism are applied to individuals in their clinical role, their relationship with their patients, and their obligations to the healthcare system. Professionalism is about aspiring to, pursuing, and meeting standards. The standards proposed in this book are accountability, altruism, duty, honor, integrity, excellence, and respect for others. In addition, one needs to be sensitive to professional obligations in a situation, be motivated to act professionally, exhibit professional judgment, and have the skills and knowledge to implement professional choices. The same standards apply to individuals in their work role within the healthcare system. For example, in your role as a supervisor, in your relationship with your boss, in the political game at work, and in personal relationships at work, the same standards hold. When acting as a supervisor (which most healthcare workers do), the standards of excellence and respect for others prevail. In other words, you should aspire to and pursue excellence in managing technicians. When you approach a situation as a supervisor, are you sensitive to your professional obligations? Do you engage in politics at work to build coalitions to improve an aspect of health care or to further my career? In dealing with your boss, do you conduct yourself as a professional? If attracted to someone at work, do you still act professionally, or do you let your emotions override your professional obligations? In reading the following sections, keep in mind your professional obligations in different circumstances.

What Are Some Facts of Organizational Life?

N O ONE IS BORN UNDERSTANDING the rules of organizational life or how to act professionally in this context. Organizations have their own rules. Here are some facts of organizational life (Data from McIntyre 2005):

- Organizations are not democracies.
- Some people have more power than others.
- All decisions are subjective.
- Your boss has significant power over your life.
- Fairness is not necessarily an organization goal.
- All organizations are somewhat dysfunctional and somewhat neurotic.

You can wish for change all you want, but these are the facts—the rules by which the game of work is played. You can choose to compete to win this game; operate as a martyr, constantly sacrificing your interests; remain clueless to the political impact of your behaviors; or operate as an amoral rogue player. The choice is yours.

Supervisors

N OT ALL HEALTHCARE WORKERS WILL be a manager. However, all healthcare workers, whether they want to or not, will act as supervisors. Any time you are working with technicians or are tasked with making sure that specific activities occur, you are acting as a supervisor. There is no grace period for assuming this role following graduation. Supervision is part of the job. It is part of being a practitioner. It is part of taking care of the patient.

Supervisors are front-line managers, interacting directly and intimately with those doing the actual work. This is in contrast to middle managers and top management who are relatively distant from the actual work of the department. As a front-line supervisor, you will be expected to engage in the basic patient care activities. Coupled with these activities is the obligation to guide and direct the work of others. If the supervisory role is more formalized, then you will be concerned with staffing, budgeting, performance appraisal, hiring, and firing, among other activities. As suggested earlier, the first day you are left alone following licensure and have technicians working with you, you are now a supervisor. As a supervisor and a professional, you will be expected to deliver good clinical care and good customer service that is financially sustainable. In other words, you are expected to make the patient better, make the patient and family happy, and make money for the institution.

A supervisor takes a group of people and attempts to direct, govern, control, steer, persuade, convince, induce, prevail upon, talk into, seduce, entice, coerce, administer, allure, beguile, force, strong arm, manipulate, compel, pressure, lead, excite, egg on, challenge, galvanize, goad, and inspire to accomplish the goals and objectives of the department. Why is this so hard? As the historian Barbara Tuchman (1981) noted, the human being ... "is unreliable as a scientific factor." Another way of saying it is that carbon based life forms are unpredictable.

As a supervisor, in addition to responsibilities for clinical outcomes, you will be responsible for levels of customer service and operational efficiencies (e.g., waiting time, quality, units produced per unit of time). Each of these aspects impacts revenues, cash flows, margins, and profits. The difficulty is maintaining the appropriate balance between clinical outcomes, customer service, and efficiency metrics. It is the challenge of the position. Those above you may applaud your effort but will only reward your performance. There is no "A" for effort.

Two Guidelines for Supervisors

Over time, as your career progresses, you will work out, through experience, what works for you as a supervisor. Two ideas may be helpful initially as you develop your own methods.

- **Reciprocity Drives Human Relationships:** It is unlikely that people will respond to you in a way that is different from the way that you treat them. This idea is based on the premise that you get what you expect. Treating people with courtesy, dignity, and respect will generally result in them treating you in the same way. This idea is particularly critical in a service business. If you want your employees to deliver superior service, you must give them superior service when they come to you with their problems. In general, an angry person will not continue to be angry in the face of a calm, reasonable response.

- **Do What Works:** Despite what you read or believe constitutes good management or what good managers are supposed to do, the only effective guide is to do what works. If what you are doing is not working, then stop it. The object is to win the game. Knowing and doing are not the same thing. Being able to analyze a case, identify a problem, or recite a correct answer is not the same as being able to effectively supervise.

What Mistakes Do New Supervisors Make?

Almost all new supervisors are prone to make two mistakes. The first mistaken tendency is for new supervisors to want the staff and employees to like them. Often, the staff and employees are contemporaries in age and experience. Often, they have shared the same work situations. In many cases, they are your friends or drinking partners. Successful supervisors have to gain the respect and trust of the people they manage. The fact that one is a superior clinician with a great track record is not enough. Supervisors gain respect and trust by first demonstrating the content of their character. As a new supervisor, employees will read every gesture and comment you make to get a handle on who you are and how you will react in this role. Will you let the title go to your head? Will you consider your employees' feelings and concerns? Will your position be about advancing their careers and aspirations or yours? Will you ask them to do things that you would not do yourself? Like a farmer searches the sky for the nuances of the weather, employees will search to get a handle on you and your style and patterns as a supervisor. Will the atmosphere at work be calm and professional or stormy, unpredictable, and chaotic?

The second mistaken tendency is the need to overcontrol. In the desire to perform, new supervisors watch everything and want all decisions to come through them to make sure there are no mistakes. Very quickly it should become apparent that no one individual can watch and manage every detail and transaction. New supervisors need to understand that their job is not to do the actual work but to build a team that will accomplish organizational objectives. Rather than building relations with individuals one at a time, the necessity is to forge a collective mentality and a sense of group that is focused on the task. Rather than watch every transaction, the successful supervisor is monitoring the group and assessing the overall performance.

The Boss

THE MOST COMMON REASON WHY people leave a job is their relationship with their boss. The key relationship you have at work, without exception, is with your boss. This single individual in many ways determines the path and trajectory of your career. If you hit it off with the boss, then that path is facilitated; but if you are unfortunate enough to clash with your boss, then many doors close. The management guru Peter Drucker observed that you don't have to like your boss, but you do have to manage him.

Certain key assumptions are useful in the process of managing your boss:

- You own 50% of your relationship with your boss.
- You are 100% in control of your own behavior.
- The way you behave toward your boss teaches him or her how to treat you.
- The relationship with your boss is one of mutual dependence.
- You are both fallible human beings.

Some people see themselves as extremely dependent on their boss. As such, they adopt an infantile posture toward their boss. They see their boss as omnipotent and infallible. In fact, the boss is, as are all humans, insecure and uncertain. One needs to recognize just how dependent the boss is on his or her subordinates. Through your actions, you can do your boss considerable harm. Bosses are imperfect. They are fallible. They do not have all the answers, and they are not the enemy.

Managing your boss requires that you understand your boss, the context in which he or she operates, and his or her pressures, goals, strengths, and weaknesses. What does your boss do well? What is his or her style of working and communicating? Does your boss like conflict or avoid it? Does your boss have any personal idiosyncrasies? You must recognize that your boss is not likely to change and that you are not likely to change your boss.

Similarly, you need to be candid in assessing yourself. What are your strengths and weaknesses? What are your goals and objectives? How do you prefer to communicate? Do you have any idiosyncrasies? In looking for points of resonance between you and your boss, the following questions are helpful.

- What are your boss's three greatest strengths and weaknesses? What are your three greatest strengths or weaknesses?
- What things do you work on effectively together?
- What are your greatest sources of conflict and disagreement?
- What is the weakest aspect of your relationship?

Understanding your boss's strengths and weaknesses, as well as your own, is the foundation for crafting a positive relationship with your boss. First, if his or her preferred work style is one of formal communication via memos and reports, then you should adjust your behavior to that style—whether you like it or not. Second, mutual expectations for one another should be explicitly declared. Typically, your boss will not do this, and it is your job to solicit this information. Third, keep a flow of information moving upward toward your boss. You may need to find a way to frame information that he does not want, such as failures and problems. Fourth, be dependable and honest in dealing with your boss; it is the only way he or she will learn to trust you and confide in you. Fifth, be judicious in your demands on your boss's time.

Although you cannot change your boss's behavior, you can shape it. For example, if you would like your boss to speak more tactfully to you in public, then every time he or she behaves in the way you like reward your boss. After a positive encounter, say something like, "I really appreciate how this meeting went. It reaffirms why I like working here." The list of benefits you can provide your boss as an employee are limited. Remember bosses are human. They want affirmation, strokes, and compliments like everyone else. So, in shaping your boss's behavior, keep the following in mind.

- Bosses like praise for their good points, like everyone else.
- Voice public and private support for your boss's goals.
- Simplify your boss's job by taking on tasks that speak to your strengths and compensate for his or her weaknesses.

- Offer to be a sounding board for your boss's ideas and problems.
- Let people know that you are proud to work for your boss.

No matter what, you will have some type of relationship with your boss. The key to a successful career is to manage that relationship. As with all relationships, a successful relationship with your boss is based on mutual understanding, respect, and benefit.

Most of the bosses you will encounter will be reasonable people with varying degrees of experience, aptitude, and insight about their job. Like all people, they will have bad days, display insensitivity, and make mistakes. However, they are most likely well-meaning people, like you, trying to do the best they can. It is likely that most of the people you work for will subscribe to theories of management based on fairness and employee participation. For some bosses, this will not be true. Some bosses may rely on fear, intimidation, anger, and rage to motivate people. They may trample on people's feelings and set impossible standards. How do you deal with such a boss? Suggestions include the following: always be prepared for meetings; work harder to demonstrate your commitment; demonstrate that you are not a pushover by calling your boss's bluff in a nonconfrontational manner; keep things in perspective and do not take them too seriously; and stick around— the longer you stay, the more your boss will trust you. A great response to a boss going into a rant is, "You seem upset. Why don't we talk later when things calm down?" A reason to tolerate such behavior from your boss is that working with this person can advance your career. As long as the relationship and circumstances advance your career goals, then tolerating the situation makes sense. If not, leaving is in order.

Politics

POLITICS IS NOT THE MARK of an aberrant organization. It is the mark of all organizations. In an ideal world, politics at work would not exist. The focus would be on building a successful organization, maximizing health outcomes, and facilitating the personal growth and development of all concerned. Unfortunately, this is rarely the case at work. Factions exist. There is competition for resources. Coalitions form to thwart other groups. Some people do not like others. All people have some level of neurotic and dysfunctional behaviors that play out in the ongoing theater of work. Some will see your competence as an asset to the business, whereas others will see it as a threat to their position. At the extreme, politics at work can be debilitating. Generally, most organizations function reasonably well despite the politics. Although you might lament the politics of work, if you want to be effective and survive and prosper at work, it is helpful to understand how to play the political game. Some examples of political tactics are as follows (Data from Zanzi and O'Neill 2001):

- Exchanging favors
- Manipulating others
- Forming coalitions
- Persuasion
- Networking
- Ingratiation
- Providing resources

What Is Prudent Paranoia?

BY THE TERM **PRUDENT PARANOIA**, we are not considering paranoia in the pathological clinical sense. Rather, the posture one should take is one of prudent suspicion. Acting from a perspective of prudent paranoia, one monitors the activities of associates; analyzes the subtext of meetings and conversations; checks for the rise and fall of one's status and reputation; and tries to understand who is in power, who is gaining power, and whose power is slipping away. In short, the prudently paranoid person is a keen and penetrating observer of the social environment in which he or she works. It is an understanding that something is always going on that may affect that person. Think of an iceberg floating across the ocean. Only a small part is visible above the water line; the bulk of the iceberg is hidden, and the hidden part is what sunk the *Titanic*. The prudently paranoid trust the dealer but cut the cards anyway (Kramer 2002).

What Are the Unspoken Rules of Work?

ORGANIZATIONS HAVE FORMAL CHARTS INDICATING where power is located and the various reporting relationships. Implicit in these charts is the formula for how things should get done (e.g., who needs to be checked with, who needs to perform a review, who needs to provide approval). In addition to these formal charts, there is a shadow organizational framework for how things really get done. Despite where the formal chart says to go, the politically astute player understands how things really get decided. For example, you may need to know that the executive assistant to the financial officer is the key to a decision because unless she is favorable to your point, she will bury your proposal; or if you really need a response from human resources, the assistant director may be the one to see, because the director is just marking time until retirement; or the pharmacist in charge is the CEO's nephew and his job is secure no matter how he performs. In other words, one needs to learn the unspoken and unwritten rules of the workplace.

What Is Political Power? How Do You Use It?

POLITICS IS ULTIMATELY ABOUT POWER and influence. Many people are ambivalent about the exercise of power. Without power, nothing can be accomplished. The grand accomplishments of any organization are because one person, or several people, had the power to get things done. The appropriate exercise of power is a good and necessary thing. Our view of power is often shaded by our agreement with the ends for which it was used.

It is highly unlikely that a recent graduate will have much power. In this case, the task is to try and influence outcomes without having any authority. A range of tactics to influence others without formal authority include the following (Data from Baldwin, Bommer, and Rubin 2008):

- Rational persuasion: using logical arguments and facts to persuade someone
- Consultation: seeking someone's participation in developing something to win their support
- Inspirational appeal: appealing to values, ideals, and aspirations to create enthusiasm
- Ingratiation: getting someone in a good mood
- Personal appeal: appealing to someone's loyalty or friendship
- Exchange: offering to exchange favors
- Coalition: seeking the help of other people, or using the support of other people to get someone to agree with you

- Legitimizing: appealing to authority or pointing out consistency with existing norms or values
- Pressure: using demands or threats

Of these nine choices, by far the most effective are an inspirational appeal, consultation, and personal appeal, whereas the least effective are legitimizing and pressure.

In playing the political game, it is good not to discount the simple power of people liking you, for whatever reason—your personal attractiveness, your pleasant demeanor, your self-deprecating humor, or your resemblance to them. It is simply easier to get things from people if they are your friends. When you couple likeability with reciprocity (supporting others, being generous with time and expertise, and doing the little things that need to be done), you have a powerful combination for organizational success.

Grapevines and Gossip

ALL WORK PLACES HAVE INFORMAL networks or "grapevines" that convey information, stories, gossip, and rumors. Some of this information will be accurate; most will be fabricated or shaded for personal gain. It is important to make sure that you are hooked into this network. Typically, the grapevine is more interested in negative information about people and events. At work, one should assume there are no secrets. Anything you tell another person is not likely to be kept secret. Few people are absolutely discreet about everything. Consequently, anything you say negative about a coworker is likely to make its way to that person, often inaccurately conveyed. If you cannot say something complimentary about a coworker, subordinate, or superior, the best advice is to say nothing at all. Gossip has the power to tarnish, or even ruin, people's careers. Information and innuendo spread by gossip is power. Rest assured that if a colleague is spreading gossip about someone else, then he or she is probably spreading gossip about you. Absorb all the information you can about the people and issues at work, but let it die with you.

Are There Ethics in Organizational Politics?

ORGANIZATIONS ARE ABOUT ACCOMPLISHING OBJECTIVES. Successful careers are about meeting personal objectives. However, that does not mean that any action can be justified as long as it furthers either organizational objectives or personal careers. There are acceptable rules to the political game. There are sanctioned and nonsanctioned activities to the political game. Examples of sanctioned political tactics include use of expertise, networking, coalition building, persuasion, image building, and superordinate goals (generating support by linking proposals to the greater good of the organization). Examples of nonsanctioned political tactics include intimidation and innuendo, manipulation, control of information, blaming and attacking others, organizational placement (controlling promotion and assignment), co-optation (merging with another group or individual to silence them), and using surrogates (working through others). At the extreme, sabotage, mutinies, and duplicity are not acceptable. The political golden rule is this: "Never advance your own interests by harming the business or hurting other people" (McIntyre 2005).

How Do I Recognize a Toxic Political Environment?

SOME ORGANIZATIONS ARE CRIPPLED BY a malicious and toxic political landscape. Such places are to be avoided; if you are already there, then leaving is warranted. A **toxic political environment** is characterized as follows (Data from McIntyre 2005):

- Power plays and power struggles predominate.
- Management egos need to be stroked constantly.
- Management personnel are only focused on taking care of themselves.
- Entire departments are at war with one another.
- Time is spent on covering yourself rather than organizational objectives.
- Gossip and backbiting predominate.
- Disagreements are personal.

Culture

ASTUTE POLITICAL OPERATIVES AND SUPERVISORS understand the organizational culture at work. **Culture** is the way things get done at work. It is the collective beliefs, values, principles, norms, systems, symbols, and habits that guide work behavior. The culture of a specific organization is a function of the history of the organization, type of employees, management style, national culture, type of products or services provided, strategy, and technology. Culture exists at three levels. The first can be seen, felt, and heard by the uninitiated observer. This level is embodied in tangible artifacts—the way things look, how people dress, how they interact with one another, company slogans, mission statements, and the things that are awarded and recognized. The fabric of the culture is represented by organizational rituals, the myths and stories that reveal the history of the organization and how values are expressed. The *expressed* values themselves are the next level. What do people say the organization is about? The third level, the deepest level, is where the unspoken and tacit assumptions reside. They are not seen or discussed in everyday interactions. These are the "unspoken rules" of work.

Culture in a healthcare organization may be described as a culture of compliance, service, collegiality, openness, excellence, justice, trust, sustainability, caring, safety, social justice, access, or quality. Although a culture may be described in one of these terms, the unspoken truth may be that it is really a culture where efficiency or profit is the unspoken subtext for everything. The point is that organizational culture is the tank you must swim in. One either must adapt to these limitations or seek a circumstance where personal and organizational values align.

Romantic Relationships

G IVEN THE DEMOGRAPHIC CHANGE IN the last generation in the healthcare profession, the likelihood of romantic involvements at work is increased. Further, the fact that most practitioners work in larger practice settings now also increases the likelihood of romantic involvements. A generation ago, more practices were smaller organizations, typically with only two or three other people. For new practitioners in their 20s, it is hardly surprising that issues related to finding and establishing personal relationships occupy much of their energy. This discussion recognizes that you simply cannot control human behavior and the human heart.

Our focus is on romantic relationships that are voluntary on the part of both people and have no societal or ethical sanctions or impediments attached. That is, both people are single and available with no coercion or significant power differences. In other words, there is no hint of sexual harassment or quid pro quo—the romantic feelings are consensual and do not violate a specific corporate policy.

In general, companies have a right to promulgate rules and regulations regarding dating at work. However, this right has to be balanced with the employee's right to privacy. Some companies adopt strict prohibitions against romantic involvement at work. Others adopt a policy that actively discourages these relationships but nevertheless permits romantic involvements. Some organizations insist that those involved in romantic relationships inform their superiors. This option is problematic if the romantic relationship is same-sex. Some companies have the parties to a romantic relationship sign a "love contract," which is essentially a document that eliminates the employer's liability. Finally, some companies avoid adopting any formal policy and rely on unwritten rules and cultural norms to handle each situation, generally involving quiet persuasion. The key is to understand what the "rules of the game" are and act accordingly.

Failed romantic relationships create potential workplace issues with legal implications. If, after the termination of a failed romantic relationship, one party acts in a manner that is unacceptable, such acts may be construed as creating gender-based harassment rather than personal enmity. Supervisors should be cognizant of such situations and should ensure that remedial action is taken. Although one may feel angry or betrayed after a failed romantic relationship at work, it is not acceptable to act nonprofessionally or, worse, outrageously.

As an employee, one should not assume that emails and Internet use on company systems is private. Someone from the company may be reading your emails. In doing so, if they discover a romantic involvement in violation of company policy, emails that are inappropriate in content, or derogatory comments regarding others at work, then action by the company may be forthcoming. Remember, do not put something in an email that you do not want others to read.

No matter how discreet one believes he or she may be, such relationships are seldom secret for long. People will notice, with some being supportive and others jealous and condemning. People will look for issues of favoritism. People will look to see whether the quantity and quality of work are impacted. People will want to know if their desires in the organization are being responded to equitably or whether they are somehow compromised by this new relationship. It is difficult to maintain a professional relationship with someone you are romantically linked to. It is equally difficult to keep it secret.

The ending of a romantic relationship is fraught with peril as well. Suddenness and the desire of one person to end the relationship can result in a messy and prolonged separation stage. Just as it is difficult to maintain a professional relationship with someone you are enamored of, it is just as, or even more, difficult to maintain a professional relationship with someone who has broken your heart. Consider 12-hour days spent next to a colleague who you have just broken up with. To say the least, it will be awkward. At the extreme, one partner's desire to maintain the relationship may become obsessive and disruptive.

The illusion of a romantic relationship is also an issue. Frequent or exclusive lunches together fuel the rumor mill and beget gossip. Such gossip, even if unfounded, may impact your reputation on the

Box 11-1 General Guidelines for Romantic Relationships at Work

- Conduct yourself as a professional. Be discrete and avoid public displays of affection.
- Do not take long lunches or breaks together. Avoid returning with a disheveled appearance.
- Love may be blind, but your colleagues are not.
- Romantic relationships with clients, suppliers, and vendors create potential conflicts of interest.
- Asking someone for a date, if company policy allows, is acceptable. Overly aggressive persistence may constitute harassment.
- Do not call in sick on the same day as someone with whom you are romantically linked.
- If working in an environment with international colleagues, recognize that different cultural norms may apply.

Source: Data from Schaefer, C. M., and Tudor, T. R. (2001). Managing workplace romances. *Advanced Management Journal.* 66 (3), 4–10.

supposition that many people believe that where there is smoke, there is fire. If there are issues with your performance, people may see this imagined relationship as contributory. There are no secrets at work. No matter how clandestine you believe you are, someone will pick up on the subtle cues. Be aware of this, and conduct yourself in a manner that does not compromise your professional reputation, your credibility, and more importantly, your performance. There is very little you can do to silence the rumor mill other than to be conscious of how your behavior is perceived.

Sexuality and Sexual Humor at Work

SEXUAL BANTERING AND FLIRTING ARE common at work, as is sexual humor. The issue is the distinction between these activities as consensual agreements between willing parties and sexual harassment. Sexual harassment is against the law. Sexual bantering, flirting, and sexual humor may be illegal if they create an intimidating, hostile, or offensive environment. Comments acceptable to one person may be offensive to another. Comments at a certain time may be appropriate, whereas the same comments in a different context may be unacceptable. If you are the object of unwarranted attention or humor, the first recourse is to confront the individual directly and convey your objections. If this does not work, then going to a supervisor is appropriate. In health care, sexual bantering, flirting, and sexual humor may be used to reduce stress. Again, this may be appropriate or not, depending on individuals and circumstances. It is important to remember the following: be aware of the norms of the workplace; evaluate the potential risk to your career; and be sensitive to the reactions of people when engaged in these behaviors.

Recall that one aspect of professionalism is the ability to implement your professional judgments and to have the courage and skills to do what is required for the patient. By acting professionally as an employee and by conducting yourself as an effective supervisor, who is capable of relating effectively with your boss, who understands the culture and political climate, and who does not let personal relationships at work impact performance, your ability to be effective is enhanced. You will be seen as someone worthy of respect, a "player" in the work game to be reckoned with.

Conclusion

THIS IS A CHAPTER ABOUT work. The chapter discusses your role as a supervisor, dealing with your boss, politics at work, and romantic relationships at work. As a professional, you are charged with implementing your professional judgments, and understanding the aspects of work covered in this chapter is relevant to that implementation.

What Do the Practitioners/Others Say?

FOR NEXT CLASS, BE PREPARED to discuss issues at work based on any *one* of the following:

- A discussion with your colleagues, or others, on how they feel and what they know about issues at work.
- An article on issues at work, either from the research literature or any other source.
- A movie, television program, or YouTube video about issues at work.
- A book on issues at work (literary, historical, psychological, or any other source).

Personal Learning Plan: Work

USE THE FOLLOWING GUIDE TO develop a personal learning plan for yourself on establishing credibility.

What prompted you to develop this plan?	
What is the general area for improvement?	
What is the specific issue for improvement?	
Why is this important to you?	
How do you generally act in these areas?	
What are your goals?	
What strategies are required?	
Who/what is necessary to meet your goals with this strategy?	
How will you measure success/failure with this effort?	
How will you reflect and capture the lesson from this effort that can be generalized to other circumstances?	

The Students: Personal and Professional Issues

BASED ON THE DESCRIPTION OF each student at the beginning of the chapter, what are the personal and professional issues (either immediately or in the future) confronting each student? Consider whether they are linked and, if so, how. Finally, what would you recommend to each student to resolve these issues?

Dana S.

Personal Issues

Professional Issues

Are They Linked? Will the Personal Issues Impact Professional Behavior?

Recommendations

Ivan T.

Personal Issues

Professional Issues

Are They Linked? Will the Personal Issues Impact Professional Behavior?

Recommendations

Niki M.

Personal Issues

Professional Issues

Are They Linked? Will the Personal Issues Impact Professional Behavior?

Recommendations

Ryan P.

Personal Issues

Professional Issues

Are They Linked? Will the Personal Issues Impact Professional Behavior?

Recommendations

Exercises

Would You Be an Understanding Boss?

Please indicate whether you think the following statements are true or false.

1. Men enjoy their jobs more than women do.

   True   *False*

2. If a worker is dissatisfied, he will produce less.

   True   *False*

3. Job satisfaction tends to increase with age.

   True   *False*

4. Men tend to rely upon their supervisors for job satisfaction more than women do.

   True   *False*

5. New employees tend to show high job satisfaction.

   True   *False*

6. Increasing workers' salaries improves their level of job contentment most of the time.

   True   *False*

7. Compared with high performers, low performers will do better if you provide them more chances to socialize on the job.

   True   *False*

8. The more intelligent a worker, the more satisfied he or she tends to be.

   True   *False*

9. Job dissatisfaction tends to increase with a worker's level of responsibility.

   True   *False*

10. Hours and work conditions are generally not important factors in job satisfaction.

    True   *False*

Scoring

Give yourself 1 point for each response that matches yours.

1. False; 2. False; 3. False; 4. False; 5. False; 6. False; 7. True; 8. True; 9. False; 10. True

A score of 5 is average. A score above 5 indicates you have a better than average understanding of what makes workers happy.

Data from Didato, S. V. (2003). *The Big Book of Personality Tests*. New York: Black Dog and Leventhal.

Discussion

1. While at work, ask your boss what he or she worries about the most. What is the hardest part of his or her job? What was the hardest thing for him or her to learn after taking the job? What was his or her strongest feeling/emotion upon accepting the position?

2. With your classmates, and based on your mind mapping exercise at the beginning of the chapter, discuss the attributes of a good boss and a bad boss. Arrive at a consensus for these traits. For this list of traits (both good and bad), rate yourself. If you are deficient in a good trait or possess a bad trait to a significant degree, discuss how you might deal with these deficiencies.

Supervision

Please read the following scenario and consider your response from an emotional intelligence/professionalism perspective. (This scenario is based on an actual event.)

The Story

Sitting at the stoplight on the way to work, at the top of the hill, MKS looked down at Larrimer Pharmacy where she worked. She looked over the small town of Steelville, situated by the Allegheny River on the edge of Pittsburgh. It was a rundown, dilapidated former mill town. Row houses and bars fronted the main streets. The best house in the city could be bought for $40,000. It looked as though the sun never shone on Steelville. It seemed to MKS that it was always cloudy on the way to work, or raining. The only buildings that reflected continued care and prosperity were the Catholic Church, the funeral homes, and Larrimer Pharmacy.

Larrimer Pharmacy was a surprisingly successful business. Entering the front of the pharmacy was like stepping into a 1950s pharmacy. MKS expected Ward and June Clever, along with the "Beav," to walk through the front door at any moment.

Business was steady in the retail side of the pharmacy, but clearly not growing. In the back, in the closed pharmacy where MKS worked, business was booming. Larrimer had contracts with two large nursing homes and was negotiating with other smaller homes. MKS attributed the success of Larrimer Pharmacy to Jackie, the nonpharmacist, third-generation family member who owned the business. Jackie was smart and tough—a real piece of work, but that is a story for a later day. MKS winced as she thought about the night she set the security alarm off and had to call and wake Jackie.

Walking into the pharmacy, MKS spotted Dave. Dave's job description is a combination technician/driver. He is an interesting young man, having gone to college to pursue an engineering degree. In his second year in school, he switched to theater and graduated with his degree. He is extremely creative, funny, and talented. He has that kind of videogame boy, slacker look; slightly disheveled, bearded, sloppy haircut, mix and match clothes, soft and fast-food pudgy. He could be thought of as an anticorporate, antipreppy, anti–Tommy Hilfiger, Nautica, Gap, and Polo kind of guy. He has a wry, cynical take on the world, as if he has just discovered that the world is not as it seems. Dave's family is personal friends with Jackie.

Some days, Dave is a very helpful in the pharmacy. On others, he is a nightmare. Today was one of those days. The pharmacy operation was designed to run with one pharmacist, two technicians, and Dave to fill in when needed. The day started badly for MKS, the pharmacist on duty. Jennifer, a board-certified technician, called just as the store opened and said she would not be coming to work. Her mother, a diagnosed schizophrenic who was constantly in and out of the hospital, had been hoarding her medications. Jennifer's mother tried to commit suicide last night. Jennifer was an industrious single mother with a small baby and a derelict boyfriend who was trying to put herself through school. MKS liked Jennifer and was worried about her.

Everything that came through the pharmacy that day was a problem. The orders were incorrect, doses were wrong, doctors were unavailable, and nurses were irritable. It seemed for every new order, the pharmacy was out of the drug, or the wholesaler had shorted the order. By 1:00 PM, orders were about 1 hour delayed from what they would normally be. It looked like MKS would have to stay an extra hour to finish everything. This was not something MKS wanted to do because she was supposed to meet someone for a drink, someone she liked and with whom she was hoping to develop a relationship. Plus, MKS wanted to make it to the mall and have a few minutes to shop for her mother's Christmas present.

MKS asked Dave to pull the Zithromax from the shelf. For a few moments, Dave broke into a splendid chorus of "It's a Small World" rendered in perfect tones and with theatrical flourish. A few pirouettes through the pharmacy, a bow, and a thank you completed the performance, which was quite good and entertaining. Dave started to pull the Zithromax from the shelf. He went to the "A" section of the shelves and started, "A, it's not here. B, it's not here. C, it's not here."

Apparently, Dave planned to go through the alphabet. MKS had just drifted to the mean side of hungry. She thought, what is this about?

Politics

Begin with a copy of the formal organization chart where you work. Construct an advice network. An advice network is based on determining who specific people would go to for advice. For example, who does the associate director go to for advice? The network should be based not on who the person is supposed to go to for advice, but who the person actually goes to. Similarly, construct a trust network. For example, who does the associate director trust with work-related concerns?

Krackhardt, D., and Hanson, J. R. (1993). Informal networks: The company. *Harvard Business Review*. July–August, 104–111.

Political Skills Inventory

Take a few moments to reflect on the following comments.

1. I spend a lot of time and effort at work networking with others.
2. At work, I know a lot of important people and I am well connected.
3. It is important that people believe I am sincere in what I say and do.

4. When communicating with others, I try to be genuine in what I way and do.

5. I always seem to instinctively know the right thing to say or do to influence others.

6. I have good intuition or savvy about how to present myself to others.

7. It is easy for me to develop good rapport with most people.

8. I am able to make most people feel comfortable and at ease around me.

Vigoda-Gadot, E., and Meisier, G. (2010). Emotions in management and the management of emotions: The impact of emotional intelligence and organizational politics on public sector employees. *Public Administration Review*. January/February, 72–86.

Romantic Relationships

Discuss the following questions with your classmates.

1. What is appropriate flirtation at work, if any?

2. What is appropriate when asking someone to go out? How persistent should you be?

3. Does overt sexuality have a place at work? Have you seen colleagues at work use their sexuality to their advantage?

4. Do people perceive these relationships differently if they believe it is the beginning of an enduring relationship or just a fling?

5. Have you observed any workplace romances? How did the people involved handle it? Were they appropriate? What were the consequences of the relationship?

6. Have you observed any nontraditional romantic relationships at work? How did the people involved handle it? Were they appropriate? What were the consequences of their relationship?

Practical Advice

Your experience and effectiveness at work is, for the most part, a function of your behavior. What follows are some practical suggestions for improving that experience, enhancing your effectiveness as a practitioner, and developing a reputation as a consummate professional.

Personal responsibility—You are in charge; no one else makes you feel or do anything. An excuse is just that, an excuse for not doing something. Although many people will applaud your effort, in general, they will only reward your performance. As one writer suggests, "Your success is your own damn fault." Although you must take credit for your setbacks, you can also take credit for your successes.

Luck—Poker players say that over the short run, luck may prevail, but over time, skill guarantees winning. Every once in a while in life, you can may be able to skate by, but over time, preparation, work, and dedication are the only things that ensure success. It has been suggested that luck is the "residue of design."

Don't confuse simple with easy—Many things in life are easy to understand but hard to do. Just because something sounds simple does not mean you can do it. Crafting a vision, creating a culture at work, motivating a tech, and using good clinical judgment are all tasks that can be understood; doing them well and consistently is another thing.

Never go over someone's head—Think about it: How would you like someone challenging your authority by going to your boss? Organizations establish reporting relationships for a reason; honor them. Only two circumstances warrant violating this caution: if your superior is doing something illegal or grossly unethical.

Stop whining—No one wants to hear it. If you need to, whine to your nonprofessional friends after hours. Better yet, tell the dog. Everyone has their own problems. Energy spent whining can be better spent just fixing the problem.

Everyone is neurotic, including you—It is easy to see it in other people, their little eccentricities of attitude and behavior or their slightly skewed take on life, work, and relationships. The Chinese say that is impossible to see your own eyelash, meaning it is difficult to see your own peculiarities because they are too close. You are neurotic like everyone else; you are just used to your neuroses.

Take the high road—If you do not know how to handle a situation, the fall back advice is to always take the high road. The fact that someone else is immature or petty does not require you to stoop to that level. Taking the high road is often the difficult choice. You might even come off second best by doing so, for now. The long-term benefit of this choice may not be apparent, but it is there nevertheless; you just cannot see it slightly over the horizon.

No one ever dies—In a larger perspective, most problems at work and in life are relatively minor, sometimes even trivial. The basketball coach Al McGuire said you only need to win two things: war and surgery. Confronted with a situation, ask yourself, "Is anyone going to die?" If not, do not get so worried. Think about how important the test that you got 88 on rather than the expected 96 is to you today or how much the date who stood you up sophomore year in high school affects you today. In short, no matter what happens, the world will continue to spin.

People are not out to get you; however, they are out for themselves—It is helpful not to see people at work as enemies. They are rivals, and like you, they are seeking advancement, awards, and recognition. Impute as high a motive to your coworkers' behaviors as you do for your own.

If it does not work, try something else—A lot of situations at work do not have easy or right answers. If the approach you are now using is not working, discard it. There are no points for style or method, only results. There are very few absolute commandments at work.

Look for the simplest solutions—If someone has trouble getting to work on time, ask the person to explain why before you develop an elaborate tracking system.

Keep things private as long as you can—Almost without exception, the way to handle any situation at work, at least initially, is privately and outside the formal mechanisms. Once memos and emails get sent, the organization has to initiate its often heavy-handed response. Few problems require a zero tolerance attitude. Situations handled in private allow people the "wiggle room" often required to save face.

Organizations are not rational places—Organizations are made up of people. People and organizations are not rational. People and organizations do stupid things; both engage in self-handicapping behaviors and both get in the way of themselves. All organizations have their inexplicable "catch-22" that does not make sense. You just have to accept this fact.

Friends at Work—People at work are not your friends. They are your professional colleagues. There is a difference. An appropriate amount of distance and circumspection in dealing with people at work is warranted.

Discuss this list with your classmates and colleagues at work and see whether they can add to this list of practical advice.

What's Important to You in the Chapter?

WITH SEVERAL OF YOUR CLASSMATES, discuss the idea or ideas that are most likely to effect change in your values, attitudes, or behaviors. Be succinct. Write no more than two sentences.

References

Baldwin, T. T., Bommer, W. H., and Rubin, R. S. (2008). *Developing Management Skills*. New York: McGraw-Hill Irwin.

Didato, S. V. (2003). *The Big Book of Personality Tests*. New York: Black Dog and Leventhal.

Krackhardt, D., and Hanson, J. R. (1993). Informal networks: The company. *Harvard Business Review*. July–August, 104–111.

Kramer, R. M. (2002). When paranoia makes sense. *Harvard Business Review*. July, 62–69.

McIntyre, M. G. (2005). *Secrets to Winning at Office Politics*. New York: St. Martin's Griffin.

Schaefer, C. M., and Tudor, T. R. (2001). Managing workplace romances. *Advanced Management Journal*. 66 (3), 4–10.

Tuchman, B. (1981). Is history a guide to the future? In *Practicing History: Selected Essays*. New York: Random House.

Vigoda-Gadot, E., and Meisier, G. (2010). Emotions in management and the management of emotions: The impact of emotional intelligence and organizational politics on public sector employees. *Public Administration Review*. January/February, 72–86.

Zanzi, A., and O'Neill, R. M. (2001). Sanctioned versus non-sanctioned political tactics. *Journal of Management Issues*. 13 (2), 245–262.

Suggested Readings

Dowd, S., and Davidhizar, R. (2003). Sexuality, sexual harassment, and sexual humor. *Health Care Manager.* 22 (2), 144–151.

Gabarro, J. J., and Kotter, J. J. (2005). Managing your boss. *Harvard Business Review.* January, 92–99.

Goleman, D., Boyatzis, R., and McKee, A. (2001). Primal leadership: The hidden driver of performance. *Harvard Business Review.* December, 43–51.

Hill, L. A. (2007). Becoming the boss. *Harvard Business Review.* January, 49–56.

Hill, L. A., and Lineback, K. (2011) Are you a good boss—or a great one? *Harvard Business Review.* January–February, 125–131.

Krackhardt, D., and Hanson, J. R. (1993). Informal networks: The company. *Harvard Business Review.* July–August, 104–111.

Kramer, R. M. (2006). The great intimidators. *Harvard Business Review.* February, 88–96.

Kurland, N. B., and Pelled, L. H. (2000). Passing the word: Toward a model of gossip and power in the workplace. *Academy of Management Review.* 25 (2), 428–438.

LeBoeuf, M. (1985). *Getting Results.* New York: Berkley Books.

Namie, G., and Namie, R. (2009). *The Bully at Work.* Naperville, IL: SourceBooks, Inc.

Scott, G. G. (2006). *A Survival Guide for Working with Bad Bosses.* New York: American Management Association.

Silverman, D. (2009). Surviving the boss from hell. *Harvard Business Review.* September, 33–40.

Sutton, R. I. (2010). *Good Boss, Bad Boss.* New York: Business Plus.

Walker, C. A. (2002). Saving your rookie managers from themselves. *Harvard Business Review.* April, 3–7.

Professionalism
as a Clinician

Preassessment: Professionalism as a Clinician

Mind Mapping

Consider the term displayed on the page. For this term, without thinking or editing, write down the ideas, concepts, examples, contradictions, and theories that come to mind. Do not arrange them in any systematic or orderly manner. Scatter them about the page. Now, draw lines between your additions indicating that there is a relationship between the terms. If something causes something else, indicate this with an arrow. Relationships may be reciprocal, meaning both cause each other, requiring arrows at both ends. Indicate the strength of the relationships by darkening and thickening the lines; stronger relationships have darker and thicker lines. **Most important: There is no right answer. Do not compare with your classmates.** *What you have is a mind map, your mental representation of these topics. Review to determine if anything has changed following this section.*

Think of what your greatest fear is upon graduation. Use that term as the center idea for your mind map exercise, for example, making a mistake and hurting a patient.

The Students

I

D ANA S. KNEW HER MOTHER only wanted the best for her. She knew her
mother wanted her to always present herself in the best light. From the
time Dana was a young adolescent until she left for school, her mother had
laid her clothes out each morning. Dana could only buy clothes with her
mother's approval. When Dana was young, her mother would meticulously
review her homework assignments and papers. This was a big part of why
Dana had done so well in high school. Dana appreciated her mother's obvious concern, but she just wanted to do something on her own.

Dana had always kept her hands and fingernails meticulously groomed.
She was lucky in that she had enough money to afford professional mani-
cures. Dana looked at her hands now; they were a disaster. She had taken to
chewing her nails. One had been chewed so much that it bled. She had also
taken to biting the skin on her hands. Lately, Dana was not sleeping. She
would lay awake at night reviewing her performance on her clinical rotations, looking for her deficiencies. Even though the informal feedback on
her performance was always positive, Dana knew her preceptors were just
being kind; they didn't know how nervous she was, how unsure she was of
her recommendations, and how frightened she was of talking to the senior
staff. Dana's performance in the didactic aspect of the program had been
outstanding. Despite all the positive feedback, Dana just knew she wasn't
that good, and she knew she wasn't ever going to be that good. At best, Dana
hoped to just barely pass the boards and find herself a job in a small, remote
practice venue where she was not likely to mess things up. Dana knew she
had just faked her way through the program.

II

Ivan T. remembered the day when he was a teenager and his father, during a drunken binge, had told him Ivan would never amount to anything,
that he would end up just like him, like all the men in the family. Ivan tossed
it off as the ranting of an inebriated, bitter man. Ivan's effort in school had
been just enough to keep him from being dismissed. He never saw himself
as being one of the elite students, even though he never had any problem

understanding the lectures or following the reasoning applied to any clinical problem.

Ivan spent most of his time looking for an angle and a shortcut. He sought out old tests, canvassed his classmates for lab results, did only the minimum on group projects, and skirted the bounds of plagiarism when writing papers. He always waited until the last minute to start projects, never sought help from an instructor if he had a bad performance, and always crammed the night before tests.

While walking across campus one afternoon, he ran into one of his professors. After a bit of small talk, the professor asked more personal questions. He said, "I see you paying attention in class. I know you get it. Do you like being in the program? Or do you regret your choice?" Ivan replied that he liked being in the program and did not regret his decision. The professor then asked if Ivan found any of the material engaging. "Yes, most of it," replied Ivan. The professor asked, "Then why is your work and performance so ragged and uneven?" The professor continued, "My sense is you have the potential for an elite residency program and graduate work if you want it. Make sure you don't regret this lack of effort someday."

III

Counting her undergraduate work, Niki M. had been in school almost 8 years straight. In hindsight, the first 4 years had been easy. The last 4 had been a struggle. She was on her own, with a son and all the attendant emotional and financial weight on her shoulders. Up until the last several months, she had handled the multiple pressures easily. She had been able to keep her focus and perspective.

For the last several months, Niki had been running on Red Bull, junk food, and 3 hours of sleep each night. It was the only way she could keep up. She was tired of winter, she was tired of having to load all of the baby's gear each time they left the house, she was tired of being alone, she was tired of not having any money, and she was worried about the upcoming clinical rotations, the impending board, and the search for a job. The last three nights, Niki hadn't slept at all. Now, sitting in her car outside her parent's house and thinking of another night alone in her basement apartment, Niki started to cry. She just couldn't make herself go into the apartment.

IV

By objective standards, Ryan P.'s life and career would be considered a success. He had a great family. There were strains and disappointments, as with any family, but overall, he felt good about how this part of his life worked out. His first career had started with Ryan going to work in the telecommunications industry as a summer intern; he had ended up in management 15 years later. The downsizing was hard to take. Initially, Ryan considered being let go as a personal failure, but with time and objectivity, he realized that he had just been caught in the numbers game that all industries go through as they mature.

Ryan felt good about returning to school. It had entailed personal sacrifice and sacrifices from his family as well. But he was going to make it; only one semester and rotations were left to complete. One thing Ryan had never discussed with anyone was the gnawing sense of failure that he carried with him every day. No matter how it looked to the outside, Ryan always felt like a failure. He remembers the day he disappointed his father. It was nothing major; he had received a "B" instead of an "A," and his father simply asked what happened. There was no yelling, and no recriminations followed. Ryan dealt with the experience by never going all out on anything again. He calculated what was just barely enough effort to perform and only worked at that level. If he went all out, he would have no excuse if things didn't succeed. If he didn't succeed with his best effort, Ryan would have to acknowledge his deficiency. The problem with his current approach is that he had no room for error.

ⅷ LEARNING OBJECTIVES

- Discuss the concept of self-efficacy.
- Discuss the fear of failure and success.
- Describe emotional labor and compassion fatigue.
- Describe worry and anxiety.
- Discuss the impact of stress.
- Discuss the concept of psychological capital.
- Discuss inner work life.

❖ KEY TERMS

- Burnout
- Compassion fatigue
- Emotional labor
- Psychological capital
- Resilience
- Self-efficacy
- Worry

Inner Work Life

I F YOUR ORGANIZATION DEMANDS KNOWLEDGE work from its people, then you undoubtedly appreciate the importance of sheer brain power. You probably recruit high-intellect people and ensure that they have access to good information. You also probably respect the power of incentives and use formal compensation systems to channel that intellectual energy down one path or another. But you might be overlooking another crucial driver of a knowledge worker's performance—that person's inner work life. People experience a constant stream of emotions, perceptions, and motivations as they react to and make sense of the events of the workday. As people arrive at their workplaces they don't check their hearts and minds at the door. Unfortunately, because their inner work life is seldom discussed in modern organizations it's all too easy for managers to pretend that private thoughts and feelings don't matter. (Amabile and Kramer 2007, p. 2)

Project yourself into the future and pretend you are on your way to work as a competent, mature practitioner when you get a phone call from your spouse. Your spouse has just come from the pediatrician, and the doctor thinks something is seriously wrong with your child. Based on the blood work the doctors order and the questions they ask, you fear that it may be serious, perhaps leukemia. It is not hard to imagine that you might be less than optimally effective at work that day. It is unlikely that anyone can compartmentalize their feelings and cognitions to the extent that the immediate concerns for the child will not be impactful. The quote above suggests, and the research on which it is based confirms, that personal inner work life impacts performance. Clinicians/practitioners are not immune to this.

In addition to the immediate circumstance described earlier, less traumatic and perhaps long buried events continue to impact a practitioner's current inner personal life. Excessive family pressures to perform, parents who fought, parents who painted a picture of strangers as menacing, or extreme childhood poverty may account for a practitioner with an inordinate fear of failure, a fear of conflict, or debilitating shyness. The resultant emotions and cognitions may result in a practitioner incapable of accepting reasonable levels of risk, confronting colleagues when warranted, or asserting himself or herself when the situation demands it. You cannot separate the clinician from the human being delivering the service. As Amabile and Kramer (2007, p. 6) note, every moment they are on the job, "employees are 'working under the influence' of their inner work lives." Prior chapters discuss how personality, emotional intelligence, and cognition and thinking influence practitioners' professional and personal growth. This chapter focuses on how the inner personal life can influence practitioners' and clinicians' work lives.

Fear and Anxiety

PEOPLE ARE AFRAID OF A lot of things, such as ghosts, cockroaches, spiders, snakes, heights, water, enclosed spaces, tunnels, bridges, social rejection, examinations, public speaking, or death. Fear and anxiety are normal reactions to potentially threatening events, either real or imagined. Individuals tend to process the world in a manner that is consistent with their beliefs about their place in the world and how the world operates. Individuals who are anxious and fearful selectively focus on events that are likely to be harmful, and even if the events are nonthreatening or neutral, they will interpret them as being dangerous. Just as a small child in his or her room believes there are goblins in the closet or under the bed and scans the ceiling for threatening shadows, excessively anxious and fearful individuals replicate this pattern in their daily lives. Fear is a basic emotion that is universal across all cultures and is hardwired into our DNA (Ekman and Cordaro 2011). The tendency to have excessive fear and anxiety tends to run in families and suggests a genetic component to this pattern. Excessive fear and anxiety are debilitating. An interesting finding is that "substantial evidence points to a preponderance of women demonstrating greater fear and anxiety than men across the life span" (McLean and Anderson 2009, p. 502).

What Is Worry?

WORRY IS THE COGNITIVE COMPONENT of anxiety; it is the anxious apprehension of events. Normal amounts of worry are beneficial. Worry is a legitimate effort to deal with and prepare for potentially stressful events. To worry about having to make a presentation during rounds is appropriate. Normal worriers attempt to refocus away from the things causing the worry. Normal worriers attempt to reframe their circumstances in such a way as to minimize their worry. In preparing to make a presentation, normal worriers might attempt to refocus their attention on some other aspect of their life once their preparations are finalized. Or normal worriers might engage in self-talk with a positive theme of, "I will do my best; that is all I can do, and they will understand that this is my first presentation and that I will improve with feedback." Normal and pathological worriers tend to worry about the same types of things. Pathological worriers, in contrast, worry about a greater number of topics, spend more time worrying, and are more likely to worry about minor things. Pathological worriers tend to focus on and look for things to worry about. Pathological worriers will see the "dark side" in any circumstance. Chronic, excessive, uncontrollable worry is central to a diagnosis of generalized anxiety disorder and is often prevalent in depression. Pathological worry is debilitating.

Fear of Failure

FEAR, ANXIETY, AND WORRY CAN be related to innumerable objects, events, individuals, or circumstances. Of particular interest to a new clinician is a fear of failure. Having never been tested in the profession, a fear of failure is appropriate. That people fear failure is intuitively obvious because failure is often accompanied by negative consequences; businesses are lost, courses and tests are not passed, spouses leave, promotions are denied, employment is terminated, and so on. The emotional consequences of failure are shame, guilt, and depression. Public humiliation often accompanies failure. Financial losses are often incurred. Hopes and dreams are short circuited, delayed, and denied. Certain fears accompany failure. Generalized fears about failure can be collapsed into the following factors: fear of experiencing shame and embarrassment, fear of devaluing one's self-estimate, fear of having an uncertain future, fear of important others losing interest, and fear of upsetting important others (Conroy 2001). Fear of failure explains why individuals self-sabotage their efforts by procrastinating or working at less than capacity. This is done to establish an excuse if they do not do well. Fear of failure also explains why individuals establish goals that are too low when compared with their potential or denigrate their accomplishments when they do succeed. Individuals high in fear of failure may exhibit behavioral patterns characterized as domineering/vindictive or non-assertive/exploitable. Fear of failure is learned, typically in a family situation that is harsh and demanding and where love is conditioned on performance. Fear of failure is linked to an excessive or neurotic drive for perfectionism. The mature response to a fear of failure is hard work. In this sense, fear of failure is beneficial.

Fear of Success

IT MAY BE COUNTERINTUITIVE, BUT many people also fear success. Fear of success is a neurotic anxiety about the negative effects of success. For the individual, success may result in social and emotional isolation, guilt over asserting oneself, a fear of discovering true potential, anxiety about surpassing an admired mentor, and a pressure to constantly match or exceed the current performance. As with the fear of failure, those fearing success will self-sabotage or self-handicap themselves to establish psychological defenses if success is not achieved. Women, in particular, may fear success to avoid the psychological tension associated with violating cultural norms and expectations. Responses to success and failure range from a success orientation to failure acceptance. The specific stages are as follows (Data from Martin and Marsh 2003):

- Success orientation: cognitively engaged and behaviorally engaged with success.
- Failure avoidance I (overstriving): beginning to engage cognitively with fear of failure but behaviorally engaged with success.
- Failure avoidance II (defensive pessimism): cognitively engaged with fear of failure and beginning to be behaviorally engaged with fear of failure.

- Failure avoidance II (self-handicapping): cognitively engaged with fear of failure and behaviorally engaged with fear of failure.
- Failure acceptance (learned helplessness): cognitively disengaged and behaviorally disengaged from fear of failure and success.

Those engaged with success are optimistic, have a belief and confidence in their ability, believe they are in control, have a focus on learning from mistakes, and are resilient in the face of setbacks. Those seeking to avoid failure are uncertain about their abilities to avoid failure and achieve success, do not believe they are in control, are not resilient in the face of setbacks, and may sabotage their chance for success. Those who accept failure have simply given up, lacking both motivation and resilience.

Emotional Labor

CONSUMERS AND PATIENTS EVALUATE SERVICE encounters based not only on the reliability and timeliness of the service, but also on the emotions displayed by the service provider. Was the waitress friendly, the ticket taker pleasant, or the pharmacist empathic? Could I, as the consumer, feel that the pharmacist cared about me and my circumstances? When I conveyed my situation, was the reaction appropriate and was it genuine? For a few moments, could I feel that the practitioner cared about me, or did I sense I was an interruption? Did the practitioner smile when appropriate, furl his or her eyebrows at the right point, and seem saddened by my loss? Service jobs, in general, and healthcare jobs, in particular, require people to regulate their emotions to fit the circumstances. The original work in this field, *The Managed Heart* (Hochschild 2012), captured this idea. This emotional requirement is termed emotional labor. **Emotional labor** is when feelings are changed or masked based on specific organizational requirements.

In any situation, the healthcare provider's emotional state may be either congruent (felt and expressed emotions may be consistent) or discordant (felt and expressed emotions are different). Two emotional labor strategies result in congruent emotional states. Those strategies are:

- **Deep acting:** In deep acting, the individual internalizes the required emotional reaction. Initially the individual may have to modify his or her felt emotions so that what is presented on the outside matches what is inside. There may be an initial discordance, but with the investment of time and energy, this discordance is resolved. Think of someone initially repelled by a class of patients who grows to care for them and displays that concern.

- **Emotional consonance:** The individual's natural emotions are in line with what is expected. Generally, individuals have a natural affinity and compassion for small babies, thus displaying the appropriate emotional reactions is genuine.

One emotional labor strategy results in a discordant emotional state. That strategy is:

- **Surface acting:** This is presenting a façade or putting on a mask because what is shown is what is expected. With surface acting, true emotions are not modified. Think of having to act polite and concerned while a patient rants and raves at you. With surface acting, the emotional dissonance is never resolved. Alternatively, the emotions may simply be suppressed.

In meeting the "feeling rules" for the situation, practitioners may have to suppress their anxiety, anger, fear, and dislike to display calm, kindness, and empathy. Over time, emotional dissonance may become debilitating, leading to both physiological and psychological problems.

Emotional labor, particularly when dissonant, may lead to burnout, affect job satisfaction, cause intent to leave, and negatively impact performance. Those who engage in surface acting without ever resolving the tension between felt and required emotions are most likely to experience these negative consequences.

Compassion Fatigue

"COMPASSION FATIGUE DESCRIBES THE EMOTIONAL, physical, social, and spiritual exhaustion that overtakes a person and causes a pervasive decline in his or her desire, ability, and energy to feel and care for others" (McHolm 2006, p. 12). **Compassion fatigue** is a result of helping others in distress. As a result, the caregiver is traumatized. Compassion fatigue is similar to burnout. Burnout is progressive and results in indifference, disengagement, and withdrawal. Compassion fatigue is sometimes acute in onset, although the underlying stresses often build over time and may result in over involvement with the patient. Compassion fatigue is often character-ized by a sense of helplessness and confusion. Compassion fatigue is the result of high levels of involvement with a patient without the compensating reward of seeing improvement. Practitioners involved with end-of-life care would be likely candidates to suffer compassion fatigue. The symptoms of compassion fatigue are as follows (Data from Lombardo and Eyre 2011):

- **Work related:** Avoidance or dread of working with certain patients; reduced ability to feel empathy toward patients or families; frequent use of sick days; lack of joyfulness
- **Physical:** Headaches, digestive problems, muscle tension, sleep dis-turbances, fatigue, cardiac symptoms
- **Emotional:** Mood swings, restlessness, irritability, oversensitivity, anxiety, depression, anger and resentment, loss of objectivity, mem-ory issues, excessive use of alcohol, nicotine, and illicit drugs, and poor concentration, focus, and judgment

Although any single symptom may indicate compassion fatigue, generally more than one symptom is required to confirm this assessment.

Burnout

THE DEVELOPMENT OF **BURNOUT** IS often insidious. It is similar to a frog in a beaker of water where the temperature gradually rises so that the frog does not realize it is being boiled. Burnout involves the loss of idealism, energy, and purpose. In burnout, mental and physical resources are gradu-ally depleted. Different levels of burnout may develop. First-level burnout is relatively mild, transient, and occasional. Second-level burnout is more stable, lasts longer, and is more difficult to eradicate. Third-level burnout is characterized by symptoms that are chronic and accompanied by a physical illness. All health professionals suffer first-level burnout during the course of a year; most experience second-level burnout sometimes, and a few move on to level three. Those experiencing burnout often attribute this feeling to a personal deficiency and feel that something must be wrong with them.

A key psychological point regarding burnout is to recognize that no matter what goes on around you, you ultimately control your response to it. A feel-ing of powerlessness is a critical contributor to burnout. Beyond this, the key recommendation for dealing with burnout is balance, primarily the balance in taking care of the patient and taking care of yourself. The same balance extends to your personal life. Your professional obligation demands that you give *of* yourself. Your professional obligation also demands that you give *to* yourself. Without the appropriate level of giving to yourself, patient care suffers.

Balance can be summarized as a blend of compassion and objectivity characterized by detached concern. There is an appropriate level of involvement. Being close allows the practitioner to see the patient as a fellow human being rather than a statistic. Being objective allows the practitioner to bring intellectual powers and professional insight to bear devoid of emotional bias. Being distant allows the practitioner to see the patient as a case. The shrewd clinician maintains the appropriate balance of each, and moves from one to the other as required.

The ultimate question is: Who will help the helper? Although help is often available at some level from various sources, the point to remember is that, most often, you will be your own helper.

Stress and Quality of Life

STRESS IS THE BODY'S REACTION to any demand. In other words, it is a response to something happening in the environment. Stress at work is due to such things as work load, lack of control, and uncertainty as to what is required. Stress is related to job satisfaction, intent to leave, and absenteeism. Workplace stress also has physiological effects such as high blood pressure, fatigue, insomnia, and headaches. In short, workplace stress is a significant contributor to whether or not a job is satisfying. It is not a question of whether there will be stress, but when and what toll will it take. The key impediment to dealing with stress is denial. Realizing that self-care is not a waste of time or a sign of weakness is the next step.

Suggestions for self-care and self-comfort follow (Data from Dahlqvist, Soderberg, and Norberg 2008):

- **Unload** by getting things "off your chest." Have the courage to admit your fears and vulnerabilities and the things that frustrate you and anger you in a safe, private environment.
- **Distract** yourself with other activities, such as exercises, reading, or watching movies, not to the point of avoidance, but to create a brief space to crystallize feelings, thoughts, and options.

- **Nurture** yourself with a small treat, and focus on your needs.
- **Withdraw** from the fray for a while; disconnect the phone, avoid emails, and be out of contact.
- **Reassure** yourself of your value, worth, and contributions.
- **Find new perspectives** on the circumstance, and view the circumstance from a different angle.

Stress and Performance

STRESS ALSO HAS SIGNIFICANT IMPACT on performance. In one view, stress has a negative impact on performance because time and energy are consumed in dealing with the stress. Also, stress tends to narrow perceptions, resulting in missed information. Concern over the physiological reactions to stress also narrows focus. Another view suggests that stress is beneficial to performance because individuals respond to the increased challenges of the situation. In this view, performance suffers if the individual is not challenged, or stressed. A third view combines both perspectives, resulting in an inverted "U" response to stress. As stress increases from low to higher levels, performance increases. Beyond a certain peak level, however, performance declines as the debilitating aspects of stress emerge. For clinicians, their reaction to stress, or lack of a reaction, is an insight with implications for impacting patient outcomes. Some clinicians may find the stress of a high-volume operation intolerable, whereas others take it in stride. Some clinicians may be energized by the feeling of walking on the edge in an intensive care setting, whereas others are rendered ineffective by the high stakes and time-constrained demands of this setting. It is unlikely that any practice setting will be devoid of performance-related stress, so learning to deal with the peculiar stresses of that setting is a professional obligation.

The lessons from psychology for improving performance include the following (Data from Hays 2009):

- **Relaxation:** Many problems relating to performance under stress stem from the anxiety associated with performance. Think of how you would converse with your colleagues in a relaxed setting versus how you would converse with them as a panel discussion in front of 500 colleagues at a professional meeting. The goal is to turn down the impact of the sympathetic nervous system. Relaxation can be learned as well as trained for.

- **Self-talk:** The goal is to not talk yourself out of performing. Self-talk, such as "I will never pass this test" or "No one will accept my recommendations," is self-defeating. Self-talk is used to reframe circumstances and cast them in a positive light.
- **Imagery:** Imagery is the concept of picturing yourself accomplishing your objective, for example, visualizing yourself passing the boards.
- **Goal setting and concentration:** Establishing outcome goals is always helpful. Establishing process goals may be even more helpful; for example, stay focused and concentrate on the present and ask yourself what you have to do now.

The key point is that one can learn to overcome the debilitating performance aspects of stress. Tennis players can learn to swing out on the match points. Similarly, you can learn how to perform under the probing questions of the chief of staff on rounds or how to take a high-stakes exam and do well.

Attitude Toward Death

I T IS IMPOSSIBLE TO BE in health care and not confront the issue of death, dying, and end-of-life care. All of us have an existential fear of death, the recognition that at some point we will cease to exist. The typical defense against this anxiety is denial. Denial, at the appropriate level, is adaptive and useful. The fear of death can be broken into eight specific dimensions: fear of the dying process, fear of the dead, fear of being destroyed, fear of significant others, fear of the unknown, fear of conscious death, fear for the body after death, and fear of premature death. (Neimeyer and Moore 1994)

Psychological Capital

T HE CENTRAL IDEA OF THIS chapter is that the practitioner's inner work life impacts performance. The topics discussed (fear, worry, fear of failure, fear of success, stress, burnout, attitude toward death) present the debilitating, or negative, aspect of inner work life. To counter this perspective, the idea of **psychological capital** is introduced. Psychological capital is "an individual's positive psychological state of development that is characterized by being confident, being positive, being resilient, and persevering in the face of adversity" (Luthans, Youssef, and Avolio 2007, p. 3). In other words, psychological capital is a framework for negating the debilitating aspects of the topics discussed and their negative impact on professional growth and performance.

Perceived Self-Efficacy

SELF-EFFICACY IS THE BELIEF THAT one can cope with adversity and accomplish difficult or novel tasks. It is the belief that you can do the job. If you do not believe you are capable of developing into a competent professional and clinician, then it is unlikely you ever will. Personal self-efficacy is a self-appraisal of one's capabilities. Personal self-efficacy derives from four sources: (1) having been successful in other aspects of your life (in short, success enhances self-efficacy); (2) vicarious experience (if they can do it, then so can I); (3) encouragement from others about your ability; and (4) emotional and physiological factors (if I am nervous with butterflies in my stomach before meeting a stranger, then I must not be good at it). Individuals have a generalized sense of self-efficacy about themselves (their global assessment of themselves) and specific self-efficacy assessments. For others to believe you are competent, you must first believe it about yourself.

Resilience

RESILIENCE IS THE ABILITY TO respond to both acute and chronic stress in a manner that is effective. Those responses are cognitive, emotional, and behavioral. Resilience is the ability to "keep on keeping on." Resilience is not a quality of the few; rather, its practice is within the grasp of everyone. Attitude is at the heart of resilience. The intent to remain in control, to persevere, to overcome, and to win is the key. The specific strengths that underlie resilience are high frustration tolerance, self-acceptance, self-belief, humor, problem solving skills, and the ability to find meaning (Data from Neenan 2009).

Hope and Optimism

HOPE AND OPTIMISM ARE COGNITIVE, emotional, and motivational estimates of the future. Hope and optimism include the ideas that good
things will occur, that you are motivated to pursue those good things, and
that you can act in such a way to realize those good things. Although hope
and optimism are almost synonymous, there are some distinctions. Hope is
a positive expectation that good things with a reasonable prospect of happening will occur. The dark side of hope is "blind hope," the delusion regarding outcomes with no chance of happening. Hope also includes the idea of
agency, that positive events are facilitated by one's personal efforts and that
one can impact events. Optimism can be thought of as a personality variable, a relatively fixed aspect of oneself. Optimists see life as a series of goals
to be accomplished and regulate their behavior to accomplish those goals.
Confronted with difficulties in pursuit of those goals, optimists persevere,
whereas pessimists withdraw.

Errors

IN THE HOSPITAL, PATIENTS ARE probably subjected to one error a day.
Most of these are not harmful. However, at least 1.5 million Americans are injured every year by medication errors. American Nurse Today
reported that there were 7,000 fatal medication errors in 2008. Approximately 4 billion prescriptions are filled annually in the United States. Even
at an error rate of one in a million, 4,000 errors occur. These statistics are for
the tangible activity of prescribing, dispensing, and administering medication. Errors in judgment are harder to quantify, as are errors in dealing with
patients. Our focus is on the emotional consequences of those errors and
the professional obligations attached to those errors.

Reactions to Errors

Think of your worst performance on an examination, report, or presentation while in school. Then think of a particularly embarrassing moment
from your life, such as something you should not have said or an inappropriate act. Now, marry the feelings associated with both. Also, think of

having to stand in front of your classmates, friends, and family and let them review your performance in both instances. Finally, the local school paper and the informal student grapevine will be abuzz with comments on what happened, how you handled the circumstances, and what it means for your graduation. The point is to have you consider what your likely emotional reaction will be to an error.

One physician likens the emotional impact of a medical error to entering "the heart of darkness" (Chirstensen, Levinson, and Dunn 1992). Errors create a cognitive dissonance for the individual between their self-image as a well-trained, competent professional whose primary goal is to improve patients' lives and someone who has harmed a patient. Errors evoke a wide array of emotional responses, including distress, panic, fear, anger, guilt, shame, humiliation, shock, embarrassment, frustration, grief, excitability, anxiety, and depression. Often these emotional reactions bleed into the practitioner's personal life. These feelings may persist for months and years. Some feelings may never completely disappear because there may be a felt need to continue to punish oneself for the transgression. Self-doubt and loss of confidence are a common psychological residue of an error. At work, relationships with colleagues may be altered. Irritability and curtness in relating to colleagues may occur. Professional reputations are tarnished. Hypervigilance, loss of confidence, and second guessing in performing work-related tasks are likely. Changes in appetite, sleep patterns, and concentration are possible. The intensity of these reactions is generally correlated with the severity of the error. Finally, there is some evidence that for significant errors women report more stress than men (Waterman et al. 2007, p. 471).

In one view, those who make errors are considered a "second victim" (Wu et al. 1993). As indicated earlier, there is no question that a medication error has a psychological and physical impact on the healthcare provider. The experience of the error and the aftermath tend to follow a predictable trajectory. The trajectory is characterized by the following stages.

Coping

Nurse Kimberly Hiatt administered 1.4 grams of calcium chloride instead of 140 milligrams to an 8-month-old pediatric patient. Five days later, the baby died. Given the baby's condition, it is not clear that the mistake killed the baby, but it clearly exacerbated the baby's cardiac dysfunction. Kim

Hiatt was fired, sanctioned by the state nursing commission, fined $3,000, required to take 80 hours of coursework on medication administration, and placed on 4 years of probation. Kim Hiatt committed suicide by hanging at age 50. She left two children. Hiatt's mother, a former nurse, said, "She was in such anguish. She ran out of coping skills."

Suicide is a form of coping; as is substance abuse, alcoholism, emotionally acting out, or any other reckless behavior following the trauma of an error. Each of these coping strategies is obviously dysfunctional. Categorizing suicide as a coping strategy is not meant to be facetious, but it is a way to eliminate the emotional pain.

Effectively coping with errors requires three things. First, one has to experience and work through all the emotions associated with the error. Denying or suppressing those emotions will ultimately lead to problems. Stoicism may be the ideal while at work, but late at night in your room, self-reflection is preferred. Depending on the severity of the error, there is a reasonable "mourning period" following the error. For a near miss that does not affect the patient, an evening after work dealing with the emotional aftermath may be sufficient. For a fatal error, a year may be in order. This period will vary for individuals; the point is that there should be a natural and healthy limit. If someone close to you has died, think of how long the recovery period was for that circumstance. At some point after the error, it is incumbent to "get on with it." Having felt and analyzed the attendant emotions, they need to be wrapped up and put in the emotional equivalent of the old business file. If this is not the case, and the emotions associated with the error are still too close to the surface, professional help is in order. Situational depression following an error is appropriate, but prolonged depression is a disease.

Imagine making a fatal error. Now imagine standing in front of the mirror as you get ready for work. What would you be telling yourself as you gaze into the mirror? It is this self-talk that is critical to the second stage of coping with the error. Some of the things you say to yourself will be appropriate; they will be both accurate and functional; other things you say to yourself will not be. The emotional intelligence exercise at the end of the chapter asks you to list the things you would tell yourself as you look in the mirror and then rate their accuracy and usefulness. The one fundamental thing you cannot say to yourself and still expect to successfully cope with the error is this: "I made a mistake, and I am a failure." This line of thinking is neither accurate nor helpful in resurrecting and continuing your career. A more appropriate line of thinking is something like this: "I'm a well-meaning professional who has put hours into honing my skills. For reasons, some of which I controlled and some of which I could not, an error was made. I did the best I could both before and after the error. I now recognize there are better ways to do things, which I will incorporate into my practice. I know of no way to practice, and continue to help people, where all possibility of error is eliminated." In his book about managing medical failure, *Forgive and Remember*, Charles Bosk (1979) offers the final and best way to think about errors. Ultimately, you must forgive yourself. Although a professional, you are human, and no human is perfect; but you must also remember the mistake so that it is never repeated and the lessons learned are applied to the patients you will help the rest of your career.

The final step in coping with the error is a detached and systematic analysis of the error, both from a personal perspective and a systems organizational perspective. The professional requirement of excellence demands it. Generally, for a fatal error to occur, multiple circumstances have to line up in such a way that the error gets through. In other words, most errors are caught due to professional expertise or redundant safeguards built into the systems. A specific error gets made, on a certain, day, with a certain type of patient, with the wrong drug, and the catastrophic error occurs. If any single variable changed in this sequence, the outcomes would have been completely different. It is this analysis that will ultimately bring psychological closure to the professional. Having made this analysis and improved his or her practice skills, the individual can take comfort in first meeting the professional standard, but also in understanding that the experience, awful as it may have been, was not wasted. Although one or two people may have suffered, innumerable lives in immeasurable ways will be enhanced.

Disclosure

The patient's desire for disclosure following an error is almost universal. Healthcare providers are motivated to disclose an error from a felt responsibility to the patient, to the self, to the profession, and to the community. Ethics demands that patients be informed of their health status as a result of an error. The impediment to disclosure is the impact of disclosure on the healthcare provider. Factors that impede disclosing errors include attitudinal barriers such as perfectionism, denial, and arrogance; fears and anxieties such as legal, financial, family reaction, negative publicity, and threat to personal identity; and uncertainties about which errors to disclose and how to do it.

Generally, a well-intentioned and grounded professional will work through the objections to disclosure and recognize that disclosure is inevitable. On signing the surrender document that ended World War II, Emperor Hirohito admonished his people "to endure the unendurable and suffer what is insufferable." Disclosing an error will feel the same way to most practitioners. Practitioners who suffer from an exaggerated sense of self-importance and exhibit the additional traits of a pathological medical narcissist will likely not disclose the error. Pathological medical narcissists will:

- Act in accord with an ideal self-image arising from a core of self-doubt and insecurity
- Act defensively when this ideal self-image is threatened
- Lose feelings for others as energy is devoted to defending the ideal self-image
- Exhibit a manic quest for success and achievement
- Exploit others to achieve this success and achievement
- Disown the real self that is flawed

Such individuals will attempt to rationalize or reinterpret the situation to protect themselves when disclosing the error. They will do this by using euphemistic language, distorting the consequences of the error, displacing responsibility, or making an advantageous comparison to something worse. The goal of this rationalization is for the health professional to convince himself or herself that not disclosing the error, or a less than truthful disclosure, is not morally or professionally wrong.

Conclusion

A S A PROFESSIONAL, THE TASK is to confront your fears and anxieties, your fear of success and failure, and your willingness to engage in emotional labor; recognize if you suffer from compassion fatigue or burnout; understand your attitude toward death; acknowledge your sense of self-efficacy and resilience and your ability to be optimistic; and develop your ability to cope with errors. Each of these impacts your effectiveness as a clinician.

What Do the Practitioners/Others Say?

FOR NEXT CLASS, BE PREPARED to discuss inner work life based on any *one* of the following:

- A discussion with your colleagues, or others, on how they manage their inner work life.
- An article on managing inner work life either from the research literature or any other source.
- A movie, television program, or YouTube video about inner work life.
- A book on inner work life (literary, historical, psychological, or any other source).

Personal Learning Plan: Inner Work Life

USE THE FOLLOWING GUIDE TO develop a personal learning plan for yourself on establishing credibility.

What prompted you to develop this plan?	
What is the general area for improvement?	
What is the specific issue for improvement?	
Why is this important to you?	
How do you generally act in these areas?	
What are your goals?	
What strategies are required?	
Who/what is necessary to meet your goals with this strategy?	
How will you measure success/failure with this effort?	
How will you reflect and capture the lesson from this effort that can be generalized to other circumstances?	

The Students: Personal and Professional Issues

BASED ON THE DESCRIPTION OF each student at the beginning of the chapter, what are the personal and professional issues (either immediately or in the future) confronting each student? Consider if they are linked and, if so, how. Finally, what would you recommend to each student to resolve these issues?

Dana S.

Personal Issues

Professional Issues

Are They Linked? Will the Personal Issues Impact Professional Behavior?

Recommendations

Ivan T.

Personal Issues

Professional Issues

Are They Linked? Will the Personal Issues Impact Professional Behavior?

Recommendations

Niki M.

Personal Issues

Professional Issues

Are They Linked? Will the Personal Issues Impact Professional Behavior?

Recommendations

Ryan P.

Personal Issues

Professional Issues

Are They Linked? Will the Personal Issues Impact Professional Behavior?

Recommendations

Exercises

Test Anxiety

Discuss with several of your classmates your particular strategies for dealing with test anxiety. Describe what you say to yourself before you take a test; describe what you say to yourself after you receive the grade.

Worry Log

Over the next week, keep a log of all the things you worry about and how much time you devote to worrying.

Fear Inventory

List the five things you most fear. For each fear, answer the following questions.

1. How long have you had this fear?
2. Can you trace the genesis of this fear?
3. Does it impact your life today?

What Exactly Is a Failure?

Please indicate which of the following circumstances constitutes a failure. Check the ones you consider to be a failure.

1. You are world record holder in the marathon. You come in first and miss the world record by 8 seconds. _____

2. You are a world-class runner. In a particular event, you have never finished higher than 10th. This time, you finish sixth but do NOT beat your best time. _____

3. You are a world-class runner. In a particular event, you have never finished higher than 10th. This time, you finish 11th and beat your best time.

4. You beat the age group record time (over 55) but finish in the last 300 runners. _____

5. You have never run a marathon before but finish in the last 50 runners. _____

6. You have completed one other marathon. This time, you do not finish the race. _____

7. You first ran in this race 60 years ago. This year, you come to the race to help with the organization. _____

Ask yourself whether it is a failure if you: do not get the residency you want, but get your third choice; have to take the board a second time; realize after a year that community practice is not for you and go back to graduate school at a reduced salary; get a raise, but not as much as you think; or get assigned to the committee you want, but are not named the chair. Is there a subjective element to failure, or is anything less than the best a failure?

Emotional Labor

1. Discuss with your classmates whether you ever "put on an act" to deal with clients or pretend to have emotions to make the patient happy.

2. If you are in a bad mood, can you modify your emotions to leave a positive impression with the patient?

3. Do you ever feel like you are faking it at work with the patients?

Fear of Failure: Performance Appraisal Inventory (Short-Form)

Please answer the following questions using this response scale.

−2	−1	0	+1	+2
Do Not Believe at All		Believe 50% of the Time		Believe 100% of the Time

1. When I am failing, I am afraid that I might not have enough talent. _____

2. When I am failing, it upsets my "plan" for the future. _____

3. When I am not succeeding, people are less interested in me. _____

4. When I am failing, important others are disappointed. _____

5. When I am failing, I worry about what others might think about me. _____

ITEM (1. _____ + 2. _____ + 3. _____ + 4. _____ + 5. _____) = _____ /5 = _____

Norms for College-Age Students

Percentile	Score
95	1.342
90	1.035
85	0.831
80	0.667
75	0.527
70	0.400
65	0.284
60	0.173
55	0.066
50	−0.040
45	−0.146
40	−0.253
35	−0.364
30	−0.481
25	−0.607
20	−0.747
15	−0.911
10	−1.115
5	−1.422

Conroy, D. E. (2003). *The Performance Failure Appraisal Inventory* (1st ed.). State College, PA: Department of Kinesiology, College of Health and Human Development, The Pennsylvania State University; p. 123.

Attitudes About Death and Dying

Consider the following questions. Compare your answers with those of several of your classmates.

When were you first aware of death?

How was death talked about in your family?

Has someone close to you died?

How often do you think about death?

Does religion influence your attitude toward death?

Do you want to know the exact date of your death?

Does death mean the end of life to you? Endless sleep and peace? A new beginning (e.g., life after death)? Or do you not know?

Generalized Self-Efficacy

Consider the following about yourself.

Do you always feel like you can manage difficult situations?

Are you resourceful in dealing with problems?

Even if someone is against you, do you still believe you can accomplish your goals?

1. Review the mind map from the opening of the chapter. Would you change anything following reading the chapter?

2. Write a one-page executive summary of the chapter.

What's Important to You in the Chapter?

WITH SEVERAL OF YOUR CLASSMATES, discuss the idea or ideas that are most likely to effect change in your values, attitudes, or behaviors. Be succinct. Write no more than two sentences.

References

Amabile, T. M., and Kramer, S. J. (2007). Inner work life: Understanding the subtext of business performance. *Harvard Business Review*. May, 2–12.

Anderson, P., and Townsend, T. (2010). *American Nurse Today*, March 2010, pg 24, www.AmericanNurseToday.com

Bosk, C. L. (1979). *Forgive and Remember*. Chicago: University of Chicago Press.

Christensen, J. F., Levinson, W., and Dunn, P. M. (1992). The heart of darkness: The impact of perceived mistakes on physicians. *Journal of General Internal Medicine*. 7, 425–431.

Conroy, D. E. (2001). Progress in the development of a multidimensional measure of fear of failure: The Performance Appraisal Inventory (PFAI). *Anxiety, Stress, and Coping*. 14, 431–452.

Dahlqvist, V., Soderberg, A., and Norberg, A. (2008). Dealing with stress: Patterns of self-comfort among healthcare students. *Nurse Education Today*. 28, 476–484.

Ekman, P., and Cordaro, D. (2011). What is meant by calling emotions basic. *Emotion Review*. 3 (4), 364–370.

Hays, K. F. (2009). *Performance Psychology in Action*. Washington, DC: American Psychological Association.

Hochschild, A. R. (2012). *The Managed Heart*. Berkeley, CA: University of California Press.

Lombardo, B., and Eyre, C. (2011). Compassion fatigue: A nurse's primer. *The Online Journal of Issues in Nursing*. 16 (1), Manuscript 3.

Luthans, F., Youssef, C. M., and Avolio, B. J. (2007). *Psychological Capital: Developing the Human Competitive Edge*. Oxford, United Kingdom: Oxford University Press.

Martin, A. J., and Marsh, H. W. (2003). Fear of failure: Friend or foe. *Australian Psychologist*. 38 (1), 31–38.

Mcholm, F. (2006). Rx for compassion fatigue. *Journal of Christian Nursing*. 23 (4), 12–19.

McLean, C. P., and Anderson, E. R. (2009). Brave men and timid women? A review of the gender differences in fear and anxiety. *Clinical Psychology Review*. 29, 496–505.

Neenan, M. (2009). *Developing Resilience*. London: Routledge.

Neimeyer, R. A., and Moore, M. K. (1994). Validity and reliability of the Multidimensional Fear of Death Scale. In *Death Anxiety Handbook. Research, Instrumentation, and Application*. R. A. Neimeyer, ed. (pp. 103–119). Washington, DC: Taylor and Francis.

Waterman, A. D., Garbutt, J., Hazel, E., et al. (2007). The emotional impact of medical errors on practicing physicians in the United States and Canada. *The Joint Commission Journal of Quality and Patient Safety.* 33 (8), 467–476.

Wu, A. W., Folkman, S., McPhee. S. J., et al. (1993). How house officers cope with their mistakes. *Western Journal of Medicine.* 159, 565–569.

Suggested Readings

Bandura, A. (1993). Perceived self-efficacy in cognitive development and functioning. *Educational Psychologist.* 28 (2), 117–148.

Blau, G., Fertig, J., Tatum D. S., Connaughton, S., Park, D. S., and Marshall, C. (2010). Further scale refinement for emotional labor. *Career Development International.* 15 (2), 188–216.

Figley, C. R. (2002). *Treating Compassion Fatigue.* New York: Brunner-Routledge.

Holmes, E. (2008). The role of emotional dissonance as an affective state on the emotional labor process of retail chain pharmacists. Unpublished Dissertation, University of Mississippi, Oxford, MS, March.

Kaldjian, L. C., Jones, E. W., Rosenthal, G. E., Tripp-Reimer, T., and Hillis. S. L. (2006). An empirically derived taxonomy of factors affecting physicians' willingness to disclose medical errors. *Journal of General Internal Medicine.* 21, 942–948.

Karim, J., and Weisz, R. (2011). Emotional intelligence as a moderator of affectivity/emotional labor and emotional labor/psychological stress. *Psychological Studies.* 56 (4), 348–359.

Lapane, K. L., and Hughes, C. M. (2004). Baseline job satisfaction and stress among pharmacists and pharmacy technicians participating in the Fleetwod phase III study. *The Consultant Pharmacist.* 19 (11), 1029–1037.

Lea, V. M., Corlett, S. A., and Rodgers, R. M. (2012). Workload and its impact on community pharmacists' job satisfaction and stress; a review of the literature. *International Journal of Pharmacy Practice.* 20 (4), 259–271.

Mann, S. (2005). A health-care model of emotional labor: An evaluation of the literature and development of a model. *Journal of Health Organization and Management.* 19 (4/5), 304–317.

Maslach, C. (1982). *Burnout: The Cost of Caring.* Upper Saddle River, NJ: Prentice-Hall.

Meron, A., Borkovec, T. D., and Ruscio, J. (2001). A taxometric investigation of the latent structure of worry. *Journal of Abnormal Psychology.* 110 (3), 413–422.

Mesmer-Magnus, J. R., DeChurch, L. A., and Wax, A. (2011). Moving emotional labor beyond surface and deep acting: A discordance-congruence perspective. *Organizational Psychology Review.* 2 (1), 6–53.

Mockler, R. J., and Dologite, D. G. (1999). Learning how to learn: Nurturing professional growth through cognitive mapping. *New England Journal of Entrepreneurship.* 2 (2), 65–80.

Muse, L. A., Harris, S. G., and Feild, H. S. (2003). Has the inverted-U theory of stress and job performance had a fair test? *Human Performance.* 16 (4), 349–364.

Ouiment, A. J., Gawronski, B., and Dozois, D. J. A. (2009). Cognitive vulnerability to anxiety: A review and integrative model. *Clinical Psychology Review.* 29, 459–470.

Peterson, C., and Seligman, M. E. P. (2004). *Character Strengths and Virtues.* Oxford, United Kingdom: Oxford University Press.

Reid, L. D., Motycka, C., Mobley, C., and Meldrum, M. (2006). Comparing self-reported burnout of pharmacy students on the founding campus with those at a distance campus. *American Journal of Pharmacy Education.* 70 (5), 1–12.

Rothschild, B. (2006). *Help for the Helper.* New York: Norton and Co.

Schwarzer, R., Babler, J., Kwiatek, P., and Schroder, K. (1997). The assessment of optimistic self-beliefs: Comparison of German, Spanish, and Chinese version of the general self-efficacy scale. *Applied Psychology: An International Review.* 46 (1), 69–88.

Scott, S. D., Hirschinger, L. E., Cox, K. R., McCoig, M., Brandt, J., and Hall, L. W. (2009). The natural history of recovery for the healthcare provider "second victim" after adverse patient events. *Quality, Safety, Health Care.* 18, 325–330.

Sender, J. W., and Moray, N. P. (1991). *Human Error: Cause, Prediction, and Reduction.* Hillsdale, NJ: Lawrence Erlbaum Associates.

Stamm, B. H. (2009). Professional Quality of Life: Compassion Satisfaction and Fatigue Version 5 (ProQOL). www.proqol.org.

Wharton, A. S. (2009). The sociology of emotional labor. *Annual Review of Sociology.* 35, 147–165.

Wicks, R. J. (2008). *The Resilient Clinician.* Oxford, United Kingdom: Oxford University Press.

Wicks, R. J. (2006). *Overcoming Secondary Stress in Medical and Nursing Practice.* Oxford, United Kingdom: Oxford University Press.

Wright, A. G. C., Pincus, A. L., Conroy, D. E., and Elliott, A. J. (2009). The pathoplastic relationship between interpersonal problems and fear of failure. *Journal of Personality.* 77 (4), 997–1024.

Zuckerman, M., and Allison, S. N. (1976). An objective measure of fear of success: Construction and validation. *Journal of Personality Assessment.* 40, 422–443.

CHAPTER 13

Interprofessional Relationships: Communicating and Connecting

Preassessment: Interprofessional Relationships: Communicating and Connecting

Mind Mapping

Consider the phrase displayed on the page. For this phrase, without thinking or editing, write down the ideas, concepts, examples, contradictions, and theories that come to mind. Do not array them in any systematic or orderly manner. Scatter them about the page. Now, draw lines between your additions indicating that there is a relationship between the terms. If something causes something else, indicate this with an arrow. Relationships may be reciprocal, meaning both cause each other, requiring arrows at both ends. Indicate the strength of the relationships by darkening and thickening the lines; stronger relationships have darker and thicker lines. **Most important: There is no right answer. Do not compare with your classmates.** *What you have is a mind map, your mental representation of these topics. Review to determine if anything has changed following this section.*

Wait Staff in a Restaurant

The Students

I

D ANA S. HAD HEARD ABOUT the hospital. The hospital was not for the faint of heart. It was high volume and high pressure. It was the lead teaching hospital in a major health system. World-class physicians, procedures, and research characterized the environment. If you didn't know your business, you would soon be found out. The hospital was known for its rapid turnover of staff. In the hospital, there was a core group of practitioners who had survived and prospered in this environment. Like soldiers on a battlefield who didn't bother to learn the new recruits' names because they would soon be dead, support for new staff from the core group was nonexistent. In fact, they were almost antagonistic.

Dana watched how the new hire was being treated. The new hire was foundering without much guidance or help from the staff. Dana had just recently begun to earn the trust of the core group. With her experience and their help, the job, though still stressful, was becoming easier. Dana was beginning to feel competent.

Dana now found the new hire outside the building on her break crying. She told Dana she was going to offer her resignation at the end of the day, even though she did not have another position. The new hire told Dana that her impending wedding would now be put on hold until she found another position.

II

Ivan T. did just about everything he could to avoid one of the nurses on the floor. The nurse was exceedingly difficult to work with. She knew her business but was often curt and overly blunt, as if she had little time for small talk or foolishness. One afternoon, Ivan and the nurse got into an argument on the floor over a small matter. The incident only lasted a few minutes, and in Ivan's mind, it was just a professional disagreement.

Ivan was considering going to the nursing supervisor with a complaint but wanted to think about it over the weekend. To his surprise, the nurse had already approached the nursing supervisor with her version of the incident. Ivan also found out that the nurse was threatening to file a complaint of sexual harassment on the grounds of a hostile work environment. The nurse claimed that all the nursing staff believed Ivan was surly in his dealings with them and that no one liked seeing him come on the floor.

III

Niki M. watched as one of her colleagues yelled at the technician about a mistake. It was more than a conversation about something gone wrong. The colleague was demeaning the technician, asserting his dominance and superiority. It was embarrassing.

Niki understood that sometimes technicians tended to exceed their authority and that sometimes they made mistakes; some mistakes were a result of carelessness, others were due to indifference, and others were just the result of the intricacies of the job. Niki also understood that the technicians were crucial to the operation because they processed most of the routine orders.

Niki did not know whether to intervene or walk away. This particular technician was first rate; she was extremely conscientious and thorough. In fact, she had just been accepted into a program to pursue her professional degree. Niki also knew that the offending colleague was viewed as the weakest member of the professional staff, particularly famous for supposedly having never been wrong or made a mistake in over 20 years.

IV

It was only the second week of clinical rotations for Ryan P. In his prior role as a manager in the telecommunications industry, Ryan had been the one asking the questions. He had standing and was aware of the respect he commanded. The senior resident leading the rounds was probably 29 years old but looked about 22 years old. The resident asked Ryan what the dose was for the patient they were reviewing. Ryan did not know and told the resident so. The resident proceeded to humiliate Ryan. It wasn't overt; the digs were unspoken. Ryan kept himself from retaliating but intended to talk to the resident later.

✦ LEARNING OBJECTIVES

- Discuss the different types of professional relationships.
- Discuss the bases of social power.

- Understand and discuss professional transactions.
- Discuss the three levels of difficult conversations.
- Describe scripting.

⊕ KEY TERMS

- Collaborative professional relationships
- Collegial professional relationships
- Consummate professional
- Friendly stranger professional relationships
- Hostile, abusive, adversarial professional relationships
- Professor/boss
- Student/employee
- Student–teacher professional relationships

Types of Professional Relationships

FIVE TYPES OF PROFESSIONAL RELATIONSHIPS are presented below. They are presented in descending order of impact on patient outcomes (Data from Schmalenberg et al. 2005):

- **Collegial** (equal power, trust, and respect)
- **Collaborative** (mutual power, trust, and respect)
- **Student–teacher** (either party can be the student or teacher; both parties are willing to listen, teach, and learn)
- **Friendly stranger** (little trust and acknowledgement, may be courteous but formal)
- **Hostile, adversarial, and abusive** (negativity in tone and action)

Professional relationships are subject to change. Moving from friendly stranger to student–teacher is an enhancement. Devolving to a hostile relationship is obviously not, but even these relationships can be rehabilitated. Collaborative relationships reflect working together, sharing responsibilities for solving problems, and making plans for patient care. These relationships are based on trust, respect, teamwork, and open communication. Trust derives from meeting others' expectations and knowing that the other professional has integrity. Even if a colleague is not likeable, he or she deserves respect.

An example of respect is having a colleague take your recommendation without verifying or confirming your work because it is you who made it. Open communication is the ability to say what needs to be said because the patient comes first, not egos. It is the ability to question and be questioned without defensiveness. Teamwork is the movement of collaboration from individual relationships to all professionals involved. Collegial relationships have all the features of collaborative relationships with the added dimension of equality. Equality of professional relationships rests on the understanding that each discipline involved in patient care has a unique and essential perspective.

Power

CURRENT PROFESSIONAL RELATIONSHIPS ARE A result of the history of each of the professions involved. For much of that history, there were significant differences in power and responsibility for the various professions. Variance in this power resulted in institutional subservience and dominance. Interprofessional power, as well as all social power, rests on five bases. These power bases are coercive power, reward power, legitimate power, referent power (someone who is exceptionally good at the job), and expert power (being the leading expert) (French and Raven 1959).

One person may combine all of the bases of social power, although it is not likely. In dealing with other professionals, it is critical to understand the bases of their power. A residency director may have legitimate power but very little expert power, having been off the floor for several years. In handling professional relationships, a key is understanding the power differences and the sources of power. Relating to a world-class transplant surgeon is completely different from relating to a student intern.

Professional Transactions

ONE METHOD OF CONSIDERING PROFESSIONAL relationships is to examine the nature and types of transactions between professionals. First, consider the perspectives individuals might adopt when interacting with one another.

> **Consummate Professional:** A consummate professional's sole focus is the patient and the patient's well-being. Acting as a consummate

professional is to consider the situation and the available information in an objective, unbiased manner and to arrive at unprejudiced conclusions. In a clinical situation, acting as the consummate professional is to consider: Is the information valid? Does the information apply in this case? Are clinical decisions appropriate from a clinical, ethical, and financial perspective? Personal issues and agendas, ego, insecurities, politics, and emotional distortions are absent when acting as consummate professionals. Consummate professionals are in control of themselves and recognize they are *only* in control of themselves, not any other professional. Students can act as consummate professionals by understanding their obligations and responsibilities in a given circumstance.

The Professor/Boss: Acting as the professor/boss is to act based on the idea of should and ought and that there are standards that need not be examined for validity and appropriateness and are invoked in an unthinking manner. The professor/boss thinks: This is the way it is done, why don't you know this? The professor/boss may say one thing and do something else. In other words, the professor/boss is willing to impose standards on you but cut corners for himself or herself. Much of what the professor/boss believes is appropriate. These well-structured and strongly held beliefs expedite outcomes. The professor/boss is never in doubt. The professor/boss believes he or she is in control of everything. Any problems that arise in a professional relationship are your fault.

The Student/Employee: There are two aspects to the student/ employee perspective. The first is inappropriate and may be dysfunctional. The student/employee believes he or she is not responsible for anything, not even himself or herself. The student/employee's fallback attitude is that he or she was just following the rules, the protocols, or what someone told him or her. The student/employee tends to blame others for outcomes and takes no responsibility for the consequences of his or her actions. The second perspective is positive. In this case, the student/employee is engaged in understanding how he or she might improve. The student/employee willingly defers to expertise in any form to facilitate improved patient outcomes. The 40-year practitioner committed to excellence will, at times, adopt this perspective.

All professionals exhibit aspects of each perspective over the course of their professional lives. In fact, they may exhibit each perspective in a single transaction. The key is to understand when each is appropriate. The ideal professional transaction obviously involves two consummate professionals acting with equal power and trust in a collegial relationship to positively impact patient outcomes based on objective criteria. In certain professional transactions, a professor/boss or student/employee is not just appropriate but desired. One of the professionals may in fact be a student/employee, but it is also possible that a consummate professional adopts a student/ employee perspective for a specific transaction where appropriate. Problems arise when both professionals want to act as the professor/boss; when each wants to avoid responsibility and act as the student/employee; and when one party acts as the professor/boss and the other as the consummate professional. Long-term interprofessional issues arise if one always acts from the professor/boss or student/employee mode. The point of the above framework is to provide a method of analysis and a guide for productive and nonproductive interprofessional relationships.

The above framework borrows from the work of Berne, *Games People Play* (1964), and Harris, *I'm OK–You're OK* (1969). In their work, transactions are analyzed from the perspective of the parent (professor/boss), the adult (consummate professional), and the child (student/employee). In any professional transaction, think of who is acting like the critical, controlling parent; the functioning, objective adult; and the passive and weak child.

It is important to understand that all interprofessional relationships have two aspects, the observable social aspect and the psychological aspect. The relationship may appear to be between two consummate professionals but what is actually going on is an unspoken, and often little understood, attempt to avoid responsibility (student/employee), assert dominance (professor/ boss), or defend egos (both). The point is that relationships always have a subtext that may or may not conform to what is actually said and observed. The adherence to a strict protocol by the professor/boss may be an attempt to avoid responsibility, and the powerlessness of a student/employee may be a ploy to maintain control and get you to do the work.

Communicating and Connecting

IN MANY WAYS, THE WORLD is overconnected and overcommunicated. The quest for open dialogue often leads to much noise with little insight or true understanding. What follows are recommendations for improving the communication and connection between professionals. (The focus is only on interprofessional communication. The presumption is that communicating with patients is covered in another venue.)

Why Don't People See Eye to Eye?

Two professionals consult with one another regarding a patient and the influence of the patient's family on a therapeutic regimen. Both professionals have read the same chart, interacted with the patient, and interviewed the family and come to distinct conclusions as to the best course of action. How can this be? In interacting with the world, each of us makes our own observations, which we then interpret and from which we draw our unique conclusions. Although we may each observe the same situation, we will each notice different things, attend to different cues (generally influenced by our past experiences), and apply our own unique rules to this situation. These rules have been developed and tested over time. For example, one person has learned that taking excessive risks is never warranted, whereas another believes that only he who dares wins. Finally, the conclusions and recommendations based on our unique observations and interpretation of events reflect our self-interest, that which is best or easiest for us or most familiar to us. In dealing with colleagues, to say that their position is based on their perceptions (and thus devalue) is to acknowledge the truth, just as our position is based on our perceptions. Also, we often have beliefs about colleagues that are counterproductive. For example, we may think they are selfish, naïve, controlling, irrational, or inexperienced.

Difficult Conversations

Many conversations between professionals are difficult and contentious. In any difficult conversation, it helps to understand that there are actually three conversations occurring. First, there is the "what happened" conversation. This is about attempting to get the facts right and coming to an agreement on the substance of the issue. There is also a "feelings" conversation, which is about trying to understand if our feelings about the situation are valid, appropriate, and functional. Finally, these conversations have aspects that touch our identity—our sense of competence, worthiness, goodness, being loved, self-esteem, and self-image. Conversations that impinge on our worth as a

person often escalate as we seek to defend our ego. Working through a difficult conversation requires that we suspend the assumptions that we are right
and the other is wrong, that we know the intentions of the other, and that the
other is to blame. In any difficult conversation, it is important to remember
that the only person we control is ourselves. The standard for conduct is that
of a professional who acknowledges the three levels of conversation and fos-
ters a learning conversation in pursuit of the best outcomes for the patient.

A productive learning conversation is facilitated by the following:

- Visibly tuning in to the other, establishing a robustness of presence
  and engagement by establishing eye contact, adopting an open posture, facing one another squarely, and being natural and relaxed
- Actively and empathically listening; being with the other person
  as he or she discusses his or her thoughts, feelings, behaviors, and
  experiences; and responding accordingly
- Understanding the other's point of view
- Understanding the context and background of the other's
  circumstances
- Seeking key messages and themes in the conversation, understand-
  ing the spin being applied, and discerning what is missing
- Listening to ourselves to see how we are distorting or filtering the
  conversation
- Only interrupting when it is useful and appropriate
- Using questions, probes, and summarization to enhance and clarify
- Taking time to reflect

Certain techniques are helpful in facilitating a difficult conversation with a
colleague. One is to develop a series of catch phrases for dealing with difficult
people, situations, and conversations. For example, if someone is upset, rather
than engaging with them, say, "You seem to be upset right now; let's talk later
when you feel better." Or if someone is distant and unfriendly, say, "Is there
something I have done that we should talk about?" Over time, one should
develop these fallback phrases to short circuit a conversation that is about
to go wrong and either delay it or redirect it in a more appropriate direction.

If time allows, prepare for the conversation by scripting out the various
ways the conversation could flow and preparing responses for each one. For
example, in asking for a raise, the preferred answer is, "Of course you can
have the raise you request; we are sorry we haven't given it sooner." What is

more likely as a response are comments such as: "We can't afford it in the budget." "Why do you think you deserve this raise?" "We can only give you half that much." "We can't do if for 6 months." "We can't give you an increase in salary, but we can change your title to manager." The idea is to prepare for each response or line of questioning so as not to be surprised.

Conclusion

THIS CHAPTER GIVES A DESCRIPTION of different types of professional relationships, the basis of power in relationships, and a framework for professional transactions. It discusses difficult conversations and gives an example of scripting as a method for preparing for difficult conversations with professional colleagues and others.

What Do the Practitioners/Others Say?

FOR NEXT CLASS, BE PREPARED to discuss interprofessional relationships based on any *one* of the following:

- A discussion with your colleagues, or others, on how they feel or what they know about interprofessional relationships.
- An article on interprofessional relationships, either from the research literature or any other source.
- A movie, television program, or YouTube video on interprofessional relationships.
- A book on interprofessional relationships (literary, historical, psychological, or any other source).

Personal Learning Plan: Interprofessional Relationships

USE THE FOLLOWING GUIDE TO develop a personal learning plan for yourself on establishing credibility.

What prompted you to develop this plan?	
What is the general area for improvement?	
What is the specific issue for improvement?	
Why is this important to you?	
How do you generally act in these areas?	
What are your goals?	
What strategies are required?	
Who/what is necessary to meet your goals with this strategy?	
How will you measure success/failure with this effort?	
How will you reflect and capture the lesson from this effort that can be generalized to other circumstances?	

The Students: Personal and Professional Issues

BASED ON THE DESCRIPTION OF each student at the beginning of the chapter, what are the personal and professional issues (either immediately or in the future) confronting each student? Consider if they are linked and, if so, how. Finally, what would you recommend to each student to resolve these issues?

Dana S.

Personal Issues

Professional Issues

Are They Linked? Will the Personal Issues Impact Professional Behavior?

Recommendations

Ivan T.

Personal Issues

Professional Issues

Are They Linked? Will the Personal Issues Impact Professional Behavior?

Recommendations

Niki M.

Personal Issues

Professional Issues

Are They Linked? Will the Personal Issues Impact Professional Behavior?

Recommendations

Ryan P.

Personal Issues

Professional Issues

Are They Linked? Will the Personal Issues Impact Professional Behavior?

Recommendations

Exercises

1. In dealing with a student intern, characterize an appropriate professional relationship. What is appropriate if the student intern is not performing at an adequate clinical level? At an adequate professional level?

2. What would you conclude about an individual who was rude to wait staff in a restaurant? Would you want to work with such a person?

3. Based on your responses to the two questions above, write a one-paragraph description of yourself relating to interprofessional relationships.

For the following situations, discuss with several of your classmates the "perfect" phrase to deal with the situation.

Unfriendly colleague

Argumentative colleague

Negative colleague

Bully

Complainer

Angry colleague

Micromanaging colleague

For the following situations, develop a script for the conversation to deal with them. Compare your script with that of several of your classmates.

Asking a supervisor for a reference

Asking for a higher starting salary

Giving your boss 2 weeks' notice during the peak season

Confronting a backstabbing colleague

Interprofessional Relationships and the Emotional Intelligence Framework

Using the professor/boss–consummate professional–student/employee framework described in this chapter, consider the following.

Self-aware: Which perspective do you typically adopt when dealing with other professionals or with other students on projects?

Self-management: Can you shift from one perspective to another when appropriate?

Social awareness: Characterize the students in your closest circle of acquaintances using the framework. Do the same for the professionals you associate with at work.

Relationship management: Speculate about whether there is a subtext to the most difficult relationships you have at work.

1. Review the mind map from the opening of the chapter. Would you change anything after reading the chapter?

2. Write a one-page executive summary of the chapter.

What's Important to You in the Chapter?

WITH SEVERAL OF YOUR CLASSMATES, discuss the idea or ideas that are most likely to effect change in your values, attitudes, or behaviors. Be succinct. Write no more than two sentences.

References

Berne, E. (1964). *Games People Play*. New York: Ballantine Books.

French, J. R. P., and Raven, B. (1959). The bases of social power. In *Group Dynamics*. D. Cartwright and A. Zander, eds. New York: Harper & Row.

Harris, T. A. (1969). *I'm OK–You're OK*. New York: Harper.

Schmalenberg, C., Kramer, M., King, C. R., Krugman, M., Lund, C., Poduska, D., and Rapp, D. (2005). Securing collegial/collaborative nurse-physician relationships, part 1. *Journal of Nursing Administration*. 35 (10), 450–458.

Suggested Readings

Anonymous. (2009). Fostering the pharmacist-physician relationship. *American Journal Health-System Pharmacist*. (66), 118–119.

Benjamin, S. F. (2008). *Perfect Phrases*. New York: McGraw-Hill.

Egan, G. (2010). *The Skilled Helper*. Belmont, CA: Brooks/Cole, Cengage Learning.

Hawk, C., Buckwalter, K., Byrd, L., Cigelman, S., Dorfman, L., and Ferguson, K. (2002). Health professions students' perceptions of interprofessional relationships. *Academic Medicine*. 77 (4), 354–357.

Kececi, A., and Tasocak, G. (2009). Nurse faculty members ego states: Transactional analysis approach. *Nurse Education Today*. 29, 746–752.

Lawrence, L. (2007). Applying transactional analysis and personality assessment to improve patient counseling and communication skills. *American Journal of Pharmaceutical Education*. 71 (4), 1–5.

McMahan, E. M., Hoffman, K., and McGee, G. W. (1994). Physician-nurse relationships in clinical setting: A review and critique of the literature, 1966–1992. *Medical Care Research and Review*. 51, 83–112.

Patterson, K., Grenny, J., McMillan, R., and Switzler, A. (2002). *Crucial Conversations*. New York: McGraw-Hill.

Pollan, S. M., and Levine, M. (1996). *Lifescripts*. Indianapolis, IN: Wiley Publishing.

Stone, D., Patton, B., and Heen, S. (1999). *Difficult Conversations*. New York: Penguin Group.

CHAPTER
14

Health Care in the United States

Preassessment: Health Care in the United States

Mind Mapping

*Consider the phrase displayed on the page. For this phrase, without thinking or editing, write down the ideas, concepts, examples, contradictions, and theories that come to mind. Do not array them in any systematic or orderly manner. Scatter them about the page. Now, draw lines between your additions indicating that there is a relationship between the terms. If something causes something else, indicate this with an arrow. Relationships may be reciprocal, meaning both cause each other, requiring arrows at both ends. Indicate the strength of the relationships by darkening and thickening the lines; stronger relationships have darker and thicker lines. **Most important: There is no right answer. Do not compare with your classmates.** What you have is a mind map, your mental representation of these topics. Review to determine if anything has changed following this section.*

Health Care in the United States

The Students

I

DANA S. WAS TROUBLED ABOUT one thing: what to do after high school graduation in the spring. She knew she had to make decisions about college and a career. What she really wanted to do was get married and have a family. She really liked small babies and children. She was a good student, not top level, but capable of doing almost anything she wanted if she applied herself. Dana had a cousin who was driven to succeed; her cousin was largely driven by her mother, who wanted to erase the stigma of losing the family business. Dana's cousin had just been accepted into medical school. Perhaps health care was a field where Dana could find a niche. Dana and her cousin were scheduled to have lunch this week.

II

Ivan T. went from living in a nice suburban home to living with his mother and two sisters in a two-bedroom apartment. Ivan slept on the sofa in the living room. In some ways, Ivan found this arrangement an improvement. His relationship with his mother and sisters had never been stronger as they bonded to support one another. Ivan had been a promising high school basketball player, probably a Division II scholarship player, and in the top 10% of his class. He imagined himself as a high school basketball coach. For the past 6 years, Ivan had worked as an aid in a mental health hospital to help support his mother and sisters. Ironically, Ivan, whose father was an alcoholic, was assigned to the alcohol unit and moonlighted as a bartender on weekends.

In Ivan's mind, high school had been a failure. His grades had suffered due to all the work, and he had had to quit the basketball team. Thoughts of scholarships, academic or athletic, had vanished. Ivan hated his father. He knew he would have to work his way through school. He also knew high school teachers and coaches did not make that much money. He wanted to continue to help his mother and sisters financially. Every night at work after things were quiet, Ivan would read the day-old newspapers for a few minutes. The headlines shouted about the healthcare crisis, aging populations, and Obamacare.

III

As Niki M. thought about it, she could understand why she had married her former husband. He was handsome, charming, and kind. His passion was working out, having fun, and looking good. As long as he had enough money to pay his bills, he was happy. He had no grand ambitions, but lived day to day. This was a way of looking at the world that Niki had never considered. The spring of her final year of college was glorious. The courtship with her husband had included long walks, intimate conversations, and release from the structure of maintaining her athletic scholarship and class ranking. Niki had never felt better. She still remembered how romantic their marriage was—how they eloped, got married, and spent a week in London. Niki's husband had told her he could never have children due to a childhood disease, so Niki was surprised when she found out she was pregnant. The baby was perfect, with an easy disposition and tufts of dark hair like her husband's. One day while the baby napped, as Niki dozed, she thought about how she had gone from a potential job in an elite corporation to a stay-at-home mother. The fights began 6 months after the baby was born as Niki and her husband argued over money, the future, and the requirement to provide for the baby. A few years later, Niki decided she wanted to go back to school. She needed it intellectually, and they needed it financially. It would be a perfect time as her son was entering kindergarten in the fall. Her husband thought money spent on new golf clubs was a better investment than tuition for Niki. Niki knew the marriage was a mistake.

Niki's parents were great, they let her move in to their basement with her son. They avoided telling her "I told you so" and gave her time and space to sort things out. Her parents were not ones to coddle in the face of life's adversities. Her father, after immigrating from the Caribbean, had worked his way through college. Their attitude was to get on with it. Niki knew she had to get on with it, for her sake and for her son's. She also knew that jobs for English majors were scarce and low paying and that, whatever she did, she could not leave the support of her parents. She knew she wanted to go back to school and needed a degree that would provide financial security for herself and her son.

IV

Ryan P. knew he never wanted to go through being "downsized" again. He was considering returning to school. Ryan was more of a visual, hands-on thinker than intellectually gifted in the traditional sense. High school and college had been a struggle for him. Writing papers and memorizing facts were difficult for Ryan. Math and hands-on labs were a breeze. He began to look for opportunities that would provide the financial security he craved.

⊕ LEARNING OBJECTIVES

- Discuss basic demographic trends in the United States.
- Discuss healthcare delivery in the United States.
- Discuss the economics and finance of U.S. health care.
- Discuss healthcare reform in the United States.
- Discuss the outlook for healthcare jobs in the United States.

⊕ KEY TERMS

- Strategic thinking

What Is the Value in These Readings, Statistics, and Graphs?

IMAGINE YOU ARE ABOUT TO buy your first house and you have just toured it. You ask the price, and it seems fair to you. But how do you know for sure that it is a fair price? Wouldn't it be helpful to have some comparison to other houses; to understand the history of the neighborhood; and to be able to predict the future desirability of the neighborhood? Similarly, you are about to "buy" a health profession. Wouldn't it be helpful to understand how the profession compares to other occupations and to other health professions and to understand whether the prospects for the profession are positive or in doubt? Taking a few moments to review the following readings, statistics, and graphs provides that framework and context. All choices can only be understood in relationship to something else. Further, all practitioners have an obligation to understand the world in which they practice and to be knowledgeable and informed. Practitioner decisions should be guided by clinical considerations as well as institutional and national considerations. Informed practice is a professional obligation because practitioners are accountable to society at large for their choices.

What Is Strategic Thinking?

STRATEGIC THINKING REQUIRES LOOKING AT a set of parameters, statistics, graphs, and trend lines and trying to forecast the future. It is a cold, hard, analytical look at those parameters, statistics, graphs, and trend lines unfettered by emotions and wishful thinking. It is seeing things as they are, not as we would wish them to be. The objective in this chapter is to review the demographic, economic, and financial trends in health care to provide context and to assess the impact of those parameters on the health-care discipline you are buying into.

The Prediction Dilemma

STRATEGIC THINKING IS AN ATTEMPT to understand the future and then profit from that understanding both personally and professionally. Caution regarding prediction and forecasting is in order. As Nate Silver notes, "We need to stop, and admit it: we have a prediction problem. We love to predict things—and we aren't very good at it" (2012, p. 13). In the late 1800s, if one considered the predicted rise in city populations and the fact that horse-drawn transportation was the norm, it was easy to conclude that soon major urban centers would be covered to a depth of several feet in horse dung. However, this did not happen. This is not to suggest that forecasting is a waste of time. It is not. But getting things right is difficult, if not impossible. Although some things are certain, such as the rising number of aging Baby Boomers, assessing how this ultimately impacts health care in terms of costs and quality for the next 30 years is risky. What if, for some as yet unrecognized political, economic, or social force, people in the United States increased their level of exercise and decreased their calories with the attendant shrinking in the collective body mass index, resulting in declining rates of diabetes and heart disease? Ignoring the trends is foolish, and accepting forecasts as thought of is equally foolish. G. K. Chesterton, in his book *Orthodoxy*, summed up the dilemma regarding the future and fore-casting this way: "The real trouble with this world of ours is not that it is an unreasonable world, nor even that it is a reasonable one. The commonest kind of trouble is that it is nearly reasonable, but not quite. Life is not an illogicality, yet it is a trap for logicians. It looks just a little more mathematical and regular than it is; its' exactitude is obvious; but its' inexactitude is hidden; its' wildness lies in wait."

Basic Demographics

THE U.S. POPULATION IN 2010 was 310,233,000 and is projected to rise to 439,010,000 in 2050, an increase of 42%. Two demographic trends drive much of the current situation in health care. First, the nation will continue to become more racially and ethnically diverse with the aggregate minority population becoming the majority in 2042. (Minority population is everyone other than non-Hispanic white alone population.) Second, by 2030, one in five U.S. residents will be over age 65, whereas this number was only 13.0% in 2010 (Vincent and Velkoff 2010).

Healthcare Delivery in the United States

TO SUGGEST THERE IS AN integrated national healthcare system that is managed and coordinated in the United States is inaccurate; there are multiple systems that overlap on some features. The focus of one aspect of the healthcare system is to keep people healthy—the public health system. The business of the public health system relates to the environment, water supplies, food safety, preventive health initiatives, behavioral health, and social policy. A second focus of the healthcare system is delivering medical care once people become sick. The United States spends nine times more on medical care than on public and behavioral health, despite the consistent research findings on the value and impact of healthy lifestyles. Key features that define the U.S. healthcare system include (Data from Kovner and Knickman 2011):

- The importance of institutions in delivering care: hospitals, nursing homes, community health centers, physician practices, and public health departments.

- The dominance of professionals in the system: nurses, doctors, managers, technicians, etc.
- Technology, new drugs, and electronic communication driving change.
- Tension between government control and free-market orientation.
- Dysfunctional financing and payment systems.

The major issues and challenges for the healthcare system include:

- Improving quality and eliminating errors.
- Extending access and coverage to the approximately 50 million people either lacking insurance or residing in underserved areas.
- Slowing the growth in healthcare costs.
- Encouraging healthy behavior.
- Improving the public health system.
- Improving transparency, coordination, and accountability within the system.

The stakeholders with ability to either constrain or facilitate change include:

- Consumers and taxpayers.
- Healthcare providers: doctors, nurses, hospitals, etc.
- Insurance companies, pharmaceutical companies, and for-profit organizations that sell to the healthcare system.
- The payers and those who regulate or accredit healthcare providers.

Healthcare Reform

CHANGES TO THE AMERICAN HEALTHCARE system have typically come in small increments. In 1912, Theodore Roosevelt tried to create a system of medical coverage for Americans. A significant rise in healthcare insurance occurred during World War II (WWII). Prior to WWII, only 10% of Americans had health insurance, and there was little involvement by the government in health care. Blue Cross insurance plans emerged just before WWII, and employers during the war used health insurance in lieu of salary increases, which were restricted, to attract workers. By the end of WWII, Blue Cross enrollment had increased from 6 million to 19 million. In addition, the government had the responsibility of caring for 15 million returning veterans, including 671,817 who had been wounded. In 1945, President

Truman attempted to enact mandatory health coverage that was defeated in Congress. By the mid-1950s, about two-thirds of Americans were insured by private insurance companies. Following the Kennedy assassination in 1963, President Lyndon Johnson was able to enact Medicare (coverage for the elderly) and Medicaid (coverage for the impoverished) in 1965. Many Blue Cross insurance organizations were hired to administer these plans.

Between 1967 and 1981, healthcare costs tripled in the United States and commenced an upward spiral that remains unabated today. This rise was driven by inflation; the increase in specialist doctors; more expensive technology, services, and drugs; and more expensive hospital care. During the 1990s, healthcare costs rose at twice the rate of inflation. In the early 1980s, in an effort to reduce Medicare costs, the government introduced reimbursement based on diagnostic-related groups (DRGs).

By the 2008 presidential campaign, healthcare costs had increased at three times the rate of inflation since 1970. About 15% of the population, or 46.5 million Americans, was uninsured. Premium costs per year for health insurance for a family had increased from $5,791 to $13,770 between 1999 and 2010. Fewer employers were offering health insurance as a benefit. Medicare beneficiaries had grown to about 45 million with Baby Boomers soon to enter the system in ever-larger numbers. Health care became a central issue in the 2008 election. Barack Obama won the election with 53% of the vote and carried Democratic majorities in both the House and Senate with him. The battle over healthcare reform was on.

On March 23, 2010, President Obama signed the Patient Protection and Affordable Care Act into law. On June 28, 2012, the U.S. Supreme Court essentially confirmed the constitutionality of the bill, but ruled that the expansion of Medicaid, one of the bill's provision, was unconstitutional. Health care was a central issue in the 2012 election, with Mitt Romney vowing to repeal the bill. President Obama was reelected in 2012.

The major goal of the Patient Protection and Affordable Care Act is to reduce the number of uninsured Americans. By 2019, coverage will be extended to 32 million more Americans. This will be accomplished by expanding the public/private insurance system, accomplished by:

- Internet-based exchanges in each state that will allow consumers to shop for and compare insurance policies. Rates will be kept affordable due to competition and tax credits for people with income up to four times the poverty level.

- Controls on the insurance industry, including who they must offer coverage to, what they can charge, levels of administrative costs, levels of out-of-pocket consumer costs, how to describe their policies, and the type of care they must include.
- Large employers must provide insurance coverage or face penalties. Smaller employers are exempt, but tax incentives are used to induce these companies to provide coverage.
- All Americans must have coverage by 2014 or be hit with tax penalties. People who cannot afford coverage are exempted, and tax incentives are available to help with premiums.
- Government changes how it will pay for care and the type of care it accepts as adequate. The law emphasized primary and preventive care.

The cost of the Patient Protection and Affordable Care Act is estimated to be $1.1 trillion between 2012 and 2021 by the Congressional Office Budget, or about $3,500 for every man, woman, and child in America. The true costs and projections are likely to vary from this estimate (Parks 2012).

The Economics of American Health Care

HEALTH CARE, LIKE ALL INDUSTRIES, is shaped by various economic forces. One assumption permeating much of the current debate is whether health care can be shaped by market forces rather than government intervention. To be shaped by market forces, health care needs to behave like other competitive markets. The question is whether health care is such a market. Prior to addressing this question, a minimal understanding of the four typical market structures is required. Descriptions of the four market structures follow:

- Perfectly competitive markets are characterized as having many buyers and sellers, freedom of entry and exit from the market, standardized products, full and free information, and no collusion. In such markets, allocation of resources is presumed to be shaped by supply, demand, and price.
- Monopolistic competition is similar to perfect competition. The exception is that products are not standardized and interchangeable. Price competition is minimized. Competition rests on differentiating by style, quality, or some other feature. The automobile industry is an example of this market structure.

- A monopoly is a situation with only one producer and no substitute products. This single firm controls price and supply unilaterally. A situation where there is only one buyer is termed a monopsony.
- Oligopoly is characterized by few buyers and sellers. Often a single firm dominates and exerts price leadership.

Many argue that health care is not a competitive market for the following reasons (Data from McCarthy, Schafermeyer, and Plake 2012):

- The number of buyers and sellers is maldistributed; many areas have sufficient healthcare professionals, but many do not. Suppliers are consolidating as sole practitioners disappear and hospitals, manufacturers, and suppliers merge into larger groups. Also, buyers of health care consolidate through employer groups. Consolidation increases power for the consolidating groups, but too much consolidation may eliminate aspects of competition.
- Barriers to entry are high for suppliers of health care due to licensure, certification, and accreditation requirements.
- Health care does not produce or deliver standardized products; many are customized for specific patients and circumstances.
- There is not full and free information. Although consumers may be better informed today, they still are relatively uniformed about price and quality.
- For many healthcare services, price does not matter. The demand for a life-saving procedure is immune to variations in price. No price is too high if it is your life.
- Healthcare products and services are demanded by everyone.
- Illness is unpredictable, leading to the requirement to pool risk via insurance with the attendant power accruing to the insurance company.
- Health care is seen by many as a right. The ability to pay should not preclude people from receiving health care.
- Much demand is induced by the suppliers. Physicians gain financially by ordering tests and procedures they deliver.
- Third-party insurance insulates the patient from sensitivity to price. Decreasing out-of-pocket expenses for the consumer increases demand for products and service.

Financing American Health Care

FINANCING HEALTH CARE IS CONCERNED with who pays for care, how it is paid for, how transactions are handled, and the total dollars spent on health care. Health care is not a normal commodity where consumers pay suppliers of goods and services directly. Health care differs in that the need for health care varies significantly; 20% of Americans consume 80% of healthcare dollars in any year. To deal with these issues, the United States has developed an insurance system to pay for services. Individuals and companies pay insurance premiums to insurance companies who pool the funds and then pay providers for services. Medicare is an example of public insurance, whereas Blue Cross is an example of private insurance. Figures 14-1 and 14-2 highlight and project U.S. health expenditures.

A significant change in the private insurance system was the emergence of health maintenance organizations (HMOs) in the late 1980s. HMOs use

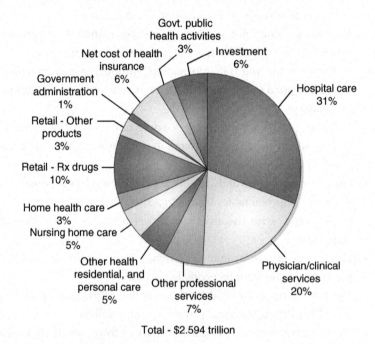

Total - $2.594 trillion

Figure 14-1   National health expenditures, 2010.

Source: Martin A. B., Lassman, D., Washington, B., Catlin, A., and National Health Expenditure Accounts Team. (2012). Growth in US health spending remained slow in 2010; health share of gross domestic product was unchanged from 2009. *Health Affairs.* 31, 208–219.

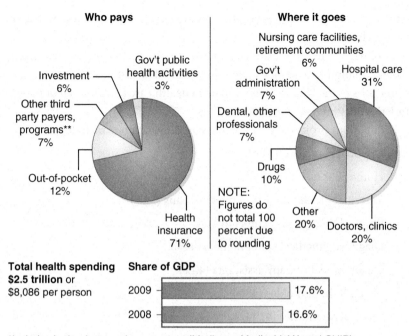

Who pays

Gov't public health activities 3%

Investment 6%

Other third party payers, programs** 7%

Out-of-pocket 12%

Health insurance 71%

Where it goes

Nursing care facilities, retirement communities 6%

Gov't administration 7%

Hospital care 31%

Dental, other professionals 7%

Drugs 10%

NOTE: Figures do not total 100 percent due to rounding

Other 20%

Doctors, clinics 20%

Total health spending
$2.5 trillion or $8,086 per person

Share of GDP

2009 — 17.6%
2008 — 16.6%

*Includes both private and government (Medicare, Medicaid, VA and CHIP)
**Includes worksite health care, workers' compensation, maternal and child health, school health, other federal and state programs

Figure 14-2   Healthcare spending.

Source: U.S. Department of Health and Human Services (2011). *Graphic:* Judy Treible.

capitated payments to control costs and control the providers in their networks. Capitated payments are fixed annual payments for each person in the HMO no matter what services are actually provided. The incentive for the HMO is to hold costs down through judicious use of healthcare services. The HMO often acts as the insurance intermediary and the provider. Despite some success in controlling costs, many consumers resent the restrictions imposed by the HMO.

The Outlook for General and Specific Healthcare Occupations

JOB PROSPECTS ARE DETERMINED BY the total population, the available labor force, and the demand for goods and services. The healthcare sector is predicted to create 28% of all new jobs in the U.S. economy between 2010 and 2020. Employment growth is projected at 33%, or 5.7 million jobs. This trend is driven by an aging population, longer life expectancies, and new treatments and technologies.

Employment in the healthcare industry is projected to increase from 14,069.2 million to 18,274.4 million between 2010 and 2020. By 2020, one in nine jobs in the United States will be in health care (U.S. Bureau of Labor Statistics 2012).

Occupations projected to have the highest growth rate include:

Personal care aides (71%)

Home health aides (69%)

Veterinary technologists and technicians (52%)

Physical therapy assistants (46%)

Diagnostic medical sonographers (44%)

Occupational therapy assistants (43%)

Physical therapy aides (43%)

Medical secretaries (41%)

Marriage and family therapists (41%)

Physical therapists (39%)

Occupations projected with largest growth in numbers include:

Registered nurses (712,000)

Home health aides (706,000)

Personal care aides (607,000)

Nursing aides, orderlies, and attendants (302,000)

Medical secretaries (210,000)

Licensed practical and licensed vocational nurses (169,000)

Physicians and surgeons (168,000)

Medical assistants (163,000)

Health Trends and Issues: Predicting the Future

HEALTH, HEALTH CARE, INNOVATION, AND human behavior are dynamic. All are constantly evolving as economic, social, financial, and psychological factors impact healthcare recipients and healthcare providers, clinicians, and administrators in different ways. One thing that can be counted on over the course of a 40-year career is that things will change. Some will profit from these changes while others will suffer. Consider the issues detailed in the following sections. What impact do you see them having on your particular practice and your career aspirations? Over the semester, keep an eye out for other issues and trends that emerge.

What if Medicare and Medicaid Costs Decline?

Innovations due to the 2010 healthcare law, less rapid development of new technologies, new drugs, increased patient cost sharing, and greater provider efficiencies influenced a $618 billion drop in projected Medicare and Medicaid spending over the next decade as reported by the Congressional Budget Office. Michael Chernew, a Harvard Medical School healthcare policy professor, believed this trend could continue (Kennedy 2013).

What if Sugar Consumption Declines?

Consumption of carbonated soft drinks, presweetened cereals, and fruit drinks and juices experienced double-digit declines in annual servings by the nation's children as reported by narcissistic personality disorder (NPD) Group. The trend "appears irreversible because the decline is only accelerating." (Horovitz 2013).

Is Obesity a Disease?

The American Medical Association (AMA) has officially recognized obesity as a disease. The declaration may influence certain reimbursement for obesity drugs, surgery, and counseling. An unintended consequence of this declaration may be to induce consumers not to care about what they consume because personal responsibility for the condition is diminished (Pollock 2013).

Vaccines

Britain is experiencing an outbreak of measles due to the failure to vaccinate infants and young children a decade ago as parents feared autism. In the United States, resistance to the papillomavirus vaccine has increased from 40 to 44% of parents declaring they did not intend to vaccinate their daughters. The virus causes 19,000 cancers yearly in women and 8,000 in men. (Editorial Board of the *New York Times* 2013; Tavernise 2013).

The $1,900 Hernia Operation

Alan Kravitz, a board-certified general surgeon, has systemized and developed a process for performing hernia operations for a flat fee of $1,900 that is targeted at the uninsured. Hernia operations take about an hour and rarely have complications. The typical charge for the procedure is $6,000 to $9,000 at a hospital. He has an assembly line process for the procedure and has been likened to Henry Ford in bringing efficiency to the procedure (Twedt 2013).

Unnecessary Procedures

American healthcare operates on a fee-for-service basis. For many practitioners, whose income is tied to the number of services provided, the temptation to overprescribe is irresistible. The end result is that, in some specialties, as much as 10 to 20% of all procedures are not warranted. (Eisler and Hansen 2013).

What Does It Really Cost?

The bill for health care in the United States is $2.7 trillion. For many procedures, the price in the United States is much higher than the rest of the world. For example, an angiogram costs $914 in the United States and $35 in Canada. Even within the United States the cost of a colonoscopy varies by city ranging from $697 to $8,577 (Rosenthal 2013).

Conclusion

THIS CHAPTER REVIEWED THE HISTORY of healthcare reform and economic, financial, and demographic factors impacting health care in America. The outlook for jobs in health care was also presented. The idea of strategic thinking was introduced as a framework for predicting and anticipating changes in health care. Several issues from current headlines were presented for consideration as to their potential impact on health care.

What Do the Practitioners/Others Say?

FOR NEXT CLASS, BE PREPARED to discuss the following:

- Discuss with a practitioner his or her observations and feelings about health care in the United States. Also, ask for the practitioner's comments and observations regarding his or her education.
- Discuss with a nonprofessional his or her observations and feelings about health care in the United States; preferably choose someone who has recently used the system.

The Students: Personal and Professional Issues

BASED ON THE DESCRIPTION OF each student at the beginning of the chapter, what are the personal and professional issues (either immediately or in the future) confronting each student? Consider if they are linked and. if so, how. Finally, what would you recommend to each student to resolve these issues?

Dana S.

Personal Issues

Professional Issues

Are They Linked? Will the Personal Issues Impact Professional Behavior?

Recommendations

Ivan T.

Personal Issues

Professional Issues

Are They Linked? Will the Personal Issues Impact Professional Behavior?

Recommendations

Niki M.

Personal Issues

Professional Issues

Are They Linked? Will the Personal Issues Impact Professional Behavior?

Recommendations

Ryan P.

Personal Issues

Professional Issues

Are They Linked? Will the Personal Issues Impact Professional Behavior?

Recommendations

Exercises

1. Similar to the characters introduced at the beginning of the chapter, prepare a one- to two-page description of yourself. Include what you believe to be the single greatest issue that dominates your emotions, thoughts, and behaviors. For example, it might be your parents' divorce or the fact that you are extremely self-conscious when meeting strangers. There is no right answer to this, and it may change with time and reflection.

2. With several of your classmates, review your decision to enter your current professional track. Was it a good choice professionally, personally, and financially? Would you recommend this track to another student?

3. Find an article that discusses the economic, financial, and social issues affecting your discipline. Prepare a one-page executive summary.

4. With several of your classmates, discuss the economic, financial, and social issues that are currently affecting your discipline and its future.

5. Are the trends highlighted in the chapter likely to positively or negatively impact your discipline?

6. Review the section on healthcare delivery in the United States. Find an article that illustrates one of the major issues and challenges for the healthcare system.

7. Review the mind map from the opening of the chapter. Would you change anything after reading the chapter?

8. Write a one-page executive summary of the chapter.

What's Important to You in the Chapter?

WITH SEVERAL OF YOUR CLASSMATES, discuss the idea or ideas that are most likely to effect change in your values, attitudes, or behaviors. Be succinct. Write no more than two sentences.

References

Editorial Board. (2013). Aftermath of an unfounded vaccine scare. *New York Times*, May 22.

Eisler, P., and Hansen, B. (2013). Under the knife for nothing. *USA Today*, June 20, pp. 1, 9A, 10A.

Horovitz, B. (2013). Is USA finally kicking its sugar habit? *USA Today*, June 3.

Kennedy, K. (2013). Medicare costs still declining. *USA Today*, May 13, p. 3A.

Kovner, A. R., and Knickman, J. R. (2011). *Health Care Delivery in the United States*. New York: Springer Publishing.

McCarthy, R. L., Schafermeyer, K. W., and Plake, K. S. (2012). *Introduction to Health Delivery: A Primer for Pharmacists*. Sudbury, MA: Jones & Bartlett Learning.

Parks, D. (2012). *Health Care Reform Simplified*. New York: Apress.

Pollock, A. (2013). AMA recognizes obesity as a disease. *New York Times*, June 18.

Rosenthal, E. (2013). The $2.7 trillion medical bill. *New York Times*, June 2, pp. 1, 18–19.

Silver, N. (2012). *The Signal and the Noise: Why So Many Predictions Fail*. New York: Penguin Press.

Tavernise, S. (2013). HPV vaccine is credited in fall of teenager's infection rate. *New York Times*, June 19.

Twedt, S. (2013). A way to beat the pain. *Pittsburgh Post Gazette*, July 7, p. 1–C.

U.S. Bureau of Labor Statistics. (2012). National Employment Matrix, employment by industry, occupation, and percent distribution, 2010 and projected 2020: Employment and output by industry, Table 2.7; Current employment survey, 2000–2010. http://www.bls.gov/opub /mlr/2012/01/art5full.pdf. Accessed August 6, 2015.

Vincent, G. K., and Velkoff, V. A. (2010). The next four decades: The older population in the United States, 2010 to 2050. *Current Population Reports*, P25–1138. Washington, DC: U.S. Census Bureau.

CHAPTER
15

Law and Ethics

Vincent Giannetti, PHD
Robert Gallagher, PharmD, JD

Preassessment: Law and Ethics

Mind Mapping

Consider the term displayed on the page. For this term, without thinking or editing, write down the ideas, concepts, examples, contradictions, and theories that come to mind. Do not array them in any systematic or orderly manner. Scatter them about the page. Now, draw lines between your additions indicating that there is a relationship between the terms. If something causes something else, indicate this with an arrow. Relationships may be reciprocal, meaning both cause each other, requiring arrows at both ends. Indicate the strength of the relationships by darkening and thickening the lines; stronger relationships have darker and thicker lines. **Most important: There is no right answer. Do not compare with your classmates.** *What you have is a mind map, your mental representation of these topics. Review to determine if anything has changed following this section.*

Ethics

The Students

I

WHEN DANA S. ARRIVED AT work, she was called into her supervisor's office. He asked her how long she had been on staff. She said since December. He showed her some invoices for materials that had been order for the office in late November. Dana didn't really look to see exactly what was detailed on the invoice.

It was hard for Dana to focus. She and one of her colleagues were working on a big project that was to be submitted at the end of the week. Her colleague had turned over her part of the work last week but what she had submitted was not usable. Dana had spent all weekend, a perfect-weather weekend, revising her colleague's work. In addition, her boyfriend was over 4 hours late picking her up for their traditional Sunday night dinner. His excuse was curious at best.

Dana's supervisor told Dana that if she would initial the invoice as having been received and date it for November, he would approve her for a big conference in Hawaii next year. Normally, to get funding for this conference, a staff member had to be an elected officer of the organization or making a presentation. Her supervisor said he had found some extra funds in the budget this year and to just sign the invoice.

II

It was ingenious and a spectacular fete of organization and secrecy. Although Ivan T. was always looking for an edge in class and at work, he never pushed the boundary. He always knew and avoided the clearly illegal. In this circumstance, Ivan wasn't sure. Would it be simple academic dishonesty, or was there a legal aspect to it? As he and his classmates graduated and began preparing for the boards, the tension mounted. The job market had tightened. Now, if you did not pass the board the first time, it meant that you would be terminated from the job. Many Facebook postings of his classmates conveyed their concern and anxiety. Even over the Internet, you could feel the tension.

From one of his friends Ivan had learned that a group of students in a southern school had been collecting test questions on the board exam and compiling them into a file. They had done it two to three questions at a time.

Each student, after taken the exam, would report back with two to three questions they had memorized. Now, more than 600 questions were in the data bank and for sale. Naturally, the sale was by word of mouth. Some of Ivan's classmates had found out about the test bank while at a fraternity brother's wedding on the southern campus. The fee to access the test bank was $500. Ivan was mulling over his choices.

III

Niki M. had a great day at the pool yesterday. It had been Father's Day. There was the traditional barbecue, and she had taken her son to the pool. They had just redesigned the pool and put in a new walk-in, gently sloping access feature. She could sit there, soak up the sun, and let her son toddle in the water. Niki was like the other compulsive mothers at the pool. If there had been SPF 500 suntan blocker, she would have used it. She spent 10 minutes making certain every nook and fold of her son's skin was protected.

Later that night, Niki sat down to go through her mail after her son was asleep. She opened the letter and couldn't believe the check—$15,000. The check accompanied the employment contract with the consulting firm she had just interviewed with. It was the sign-on bonus. A second check for moving expenses was also included. Even though they had discussed the sign-on bonus, seeing the check made the choice more real.

Rather than a clinical position, the offer was to join a big consulting firm that dealt with the insurance industry and the big integrated health systems. The initial salary for this firm was not as much as she could make in clinical practice, but the potential was greater. Over a 7-year progression Niki could move to senior consultant, then managing consultant, and finally partner. The competition for partner was fierce, but the salary and benefits could be staggering. The firm wanted a verbal commitment in their office by the end of the week and the signed contract the week after. The dilemma was that she still had another offer, a clinical offer that had been promised for later this week. It just had to be approved by the vice president of finance for the hospital. The timing for acceptance for both was very tight. Niki debated her options.

IV

While working in the telecommunications industry, Ryan was often in the field. About 18 months ago, he injured his back on the job. The company had paid for his treatment. Every once in a while, he would have a residual twinge. The pain was not debilitating, but uncomfortable. He would have to get up from his chair and stretch.

Ryan was going over the financial aid forms for himself and his daughter. He was looking to apply for as many scholarships as possible for both him and his daughter. He was amazed at the restrictions and covenants on some of the scholarship bequests that alumni had made to the schools. One scholarship was for the children of disabled parents. Ryan knew that back issues were deceptively difficult to prove or disprove. He considered applying for Social Security disability. The benefits of this were two-fold. First, he would get a considerable check for himself, more than unemployment paid, and second, his daughter would then become eligible for disability scholarship. His brother-in-law was a chiropractor who also reviewed insurance claims. Ryan believed he could help him structure his case.

⫸ LEARNING OBJECTIVES

- Discuss the distinction between law and ethics.
- Discuss the elements of negligence.
- Discuss your rights if you make an error.
- Discuss the duty to warn, nonmaleficence, informed consent, and autonomy.
- Describe an impaired professional.
- Discuss Health Insurance Portability and Accountability Act requirements.
- Describe professional boundaries.

⫸ KEY TERMS

- Autonomy
- Duty to warn
- Ethics
- Impaired professional
- Informed consent
- Law

- Liability
- Negligence
- Nonmaleficence

What Is Law? What Are Ethics? How Do They Differ? What Role Do They Play in Professional Responsibility?

Law is a body of rules, standards, and principles that the citizens of a society develop to govern conduct within the society; the observance of laws can be enforced by courts, and breaches may result in legal consequences. **Ethics** are the morally relevant criteria used to decide the outcomes of value conflicts in professional or personal judgments. Ethics may be derived from religious traditions, the social contract, or the use of reason. Evolutionary psychology has recently argued that moral intuition and ethical reasoning are traits that have been selected because of their survival value for the species.

Put simply, ethics are what one ought or ought not to do, and laws are what one must or must not do according to societal consensus based on legislative and judicial processes. For health professions, codes of ethics can have an additional force of law in that ethics violations can be adjudicated by state licensing boards in administrative hearings and sanctions applied by the board.

Healthcare professionals are governed by ethical codes, which demand a high level of integrity, honesty, and responsibility, and by laws, which regulate conduct within a profession. But the two concepts—law and ethics—do not always align. In other words, what may be appropriate ethically may not necessarily be legal, and conduct that may be legal does not ensure that it is ethical. This raises the difficult issue of conscientious objection wherein people take exceptions to law or professional duties based on a moral objection to the nature of the activity.

This also raises the issue of whether laws and regulations can be circumvented to serve a higher good. There can be times when the law does not cover all of the situations in practice. You may also find that some situations may require that you not follow the law and do what you think is the right course of action to assist the patient. In general, there is a professional obligation to follow laws and regulations that govern practice. However, if a determination is made to skirt or circumvent the law for a higher good, there are a number of conditions that should be met.

First, the decision you make must be based on an ethical principle that can be defended. For example, pharmacists giving a prescription to a patient without a prescription in an emergency situation where the patient's life could be at risk would value the preservation of life over a regulation. Second, the exception that you make to the law cannot benefit you or your organization directly, and you should not profit from the decision. In other words, self-interest should not be part of the decision. The course of action must be solely for the benefit of the patient and should be able to be defended as an altruistic act. Finally, you should report the exception and the rationale for the action to all parties involved in the transaction. There is never any guarantee that choosing to circumvent a law or regulation, even when the above-mentioned conditions are present and a higher good is served, will protect you from legal sanction. As a result, any decision to make exceptions to laws must always be the rare exception, be conducted without personal gain, involve altruism, and be documented so as to maintain transparency.

Nonetheless, law and ethics are invariably intertwined in health care. Often, answering the question of whether something is "legal" is more complicated than simply referencing a written law. Although certain laws are designed to describe the best general approach to most health care decisions, quite often they do not directly address the specific facts of a given situation. In these instances, ethical principles may provide additional guidance on what to do.

Similarly, answering the question of whether something is "ethical" is often more complicated than simply applying rules. Decision making in ethics involves understanding the relevant facts of an ethical issue, applying specific principles to the facts, deciding whether a particular ethical issue requires an exception to the principles, and deciding on what principles exceptions can be made.

Law and ethics play a considerable role in professional responsibility. A healthcare professional's "professional responsibility" essentially involves consistently exercising sound professional judgment. To exercise sound professional judgment in any given healthcare decision, a healthcare professional must know, understand, and consider the (1) law, (2) ethics, and (3) therapeutic implications at issue in the decision. Like a three-legged stool, sound professional judgment rests simultaneously upon all three of these concepts. Failure to consider any one of them when making a healthcare decision may jeopardize sound professional judgment and also the integrity of the healthcare professional's "professional responsibility" to his or her patients and profession.

This chapter will cover the basic legal and ethical imperatives that must be followed to ensure sound judgments in health care. Theories and technical terms in both law and ethics will be minimal, and the chapter does not represent a comprehensive overview of all of the possible legal and ethical issues in health care. Issues such as genetic engineering, physician-assisted suicide, end-of-life decision making, and reproductive health that are discussed in specialized courses in healthcare law and ethics will not be covered. The chapter presents relevant legal and ethical concepts that will provide guidance to sound professional judgment in common healthcare situations. Ample resources will be given in the Suggested Readings section for further reading to explore the topics in more detail. Much of the ethical and legal principles discussed in this chapter can be summarized as follows:

- Standards of care must be followed.
- Risks to patients must be mitigated.
- Patients must be informed, and autonomy must be respected.
- Professionals must be competent.
- Licensing regulations and relevant laws must be complied with.
- Patients must be treated equitably.
- Confidentiality must be respected.
- Employees should be treated fairly.
- Student loans must be repaid.
- Professional boundaries must be respected.

What Are Standards of Care, Negligence, and Liability?

IN A HEALTHCARE CONTEXT, THE standards of care help to define the level of care expected from a competent healthcare practitioner in a given practice area. Legal concepts like negligence and liability can be said to exist to hold healthcare practitioners legally accountable for the consequences of conduct that falls below the applicable standard of care.

Negligence from a healthcare perspective arises when four elements are established: (1) the healthcare professional owed a *duty* to a person to conform to specific standard of care for the protection of the person against an unreasonable risk of injury; (2) the healthcare professional *breached* that duty, and (3) the breach was the *actual and proximate cause* (4) of *harm* to the person to whom the healthcare professional owed the duty. **Liability,** which amounts to responsibility to compensate or redress for harm, only arises when all four of these elements of negligence are established.

It is important to note that negligence is not the only theory of liability for which a healthcare professional can be found liable. It is nonetheless one of the most prevalent types of liability and thus the only theory that is discussed in this chapter.

To Whom Do I Owe a Duty?

The existence of a duty is often determined by the nature of the relationship between the healthcare provider and the injured person. Not all relationships give rise to a legal duty. This helps to explain why most courts hold that healthcare providers have no legal obligation to rescue a stranger in peril, unless the healthcare provider's actions placed the stranger in harm's way. An established healthcare provider–patient relationship is, however, often sufficient to create a duty.

All of the ethical duties that are usually enumerated in codes of ethics for the respective profession and standard ethical principles apply once a healthcare provider decides to treat a patient. The implication is that for healthcare professionals there is a professional duty to take care of the patient's needs above and beyond what a routine mercantile transaction would require. The ethos of buyer beware is not consistent with health care because consumers of health care do not have the perquisite knowledge to make decisions about treatments and the risks of healthcare interventions.

How Is the Standard of Care Defined for Healthcare Professionals, and When Is It Breached?

Once it is determined that a healthcare provider owes a legal duty to another to conform to a specific standard of care, the applicable standard must be determined. For healthcare professionals, courts generally determine the standard of care by evaluating the level at which an ordinary, prudent healthcare professional with the same training and experience in good standing in the same or a similar community would practice under the same or similar circumstances. Federal and state laws, rules and regulations, and professional organizations may also help to define the standard of care.

Once the standard of care is established, a court will then compare the conduct of the healthcare professional, who is subject to a claim of negligence, to that level of conduct expected under the established standard of care. If the healthcare professional's conduct falls below that level of conduct expected under the standard of care, the healthcare professional has breached his or her duty.

Ethical duties to patients parallel legal duties. However, there are times when a legal duty may not apply, but an argument could be made for an ethical duty. If patients waive their rights to counseling or have unique social, psychological, or physical characteristics that affect their quality of life and health, then healthcare professionals should spend extra time motivating, educating, reassuring, and supporting the patient. This may not be required by a specific standard of care but would be included in the ethical duty of doing what is in the best interest of the patient. On relatively rare occasions, a professional can make a decision to contravene a law to serve a more important ethical duty. Dispensing a prescription inhaler for a patient in crisis in a pharmacy when the patient does not have a prescription may be technically illegal but ethically correct to prevent harm to the patient. These are tricky waters and require a high level of sophistication in understanding ethical principles and their application. A good place to start is to ask whether the proposed course of action is likely to result in an improved patient outcome.

What Do Actual and Proximate Cause Mean?

Actual cause means that *but for* the healthcare professional's actions the person's injury would not have occurred. Proximate cause relates to the scope of a healthcare professional's responsibility in a negligence case. It limits the healthcare professional's responsibility to only those harms that the defendant could have foreseen through his or her actions.

Here is a basic example of actual and proximate cause in a negligence case: A speeding driver collides with a truck, which injures the truck driver. The truck is carrying explosives. The truck explodes and causes a telephone pole to fall a mile down the road, which injures a bystander. Is the speeding driver liable for the bystander's injuries? *But for* the speeding driver, the bystander would not have been injured. However, it was highly unforeseeable that the bystander's injury would result from the collision. So the speeding driver will unlikely be held liable for the bystander's injuries, but he might be liable for injuries caused to the truck driver.

Here is an illustration of actual and proximate cause in a medical context: A pharmacist dispenses the wrong medication to a patient. The medication has a side effect of drowsiness. After taking the medication, and while driving to work, the patient falls asleep and hits an oncoming car, severely injuring herself and the driver of the other car. The patient then becomes depressed from her injuries and commits suicide. The pharmacist is sued for negligence because he dispensed the wrong medication.

But for the pharmacist's act of dispensing the wrong medication, the patient would not have fallen asleep, would not have crashed, and would not have committed suicide as a result of her injuries. So actual cause likely exists. It was also foreseeable at the time the pharmacist dispensed the wrong medication with a drowsiness side effect that the patient could fall asleep at the wheel while driving and cause an accident. However, it is unlikely that a court would find that the patient's suicide was foreseeable. Because both actual and proximate cause must exist, the pharmacist would likely be liable only for the patient's injuries sustained in the car crash, but not the patient's suicide. The tougher question is whether the pharmacist would be liable to the driver of the other car. Courts often struggle to answer this question.

Ethical obligations to third parties usually center on the conflict between confidentiality and risk to third parties posed by patients or other healthcare professionals. Designated informant requirements of law for healthcare professionals clearly spell out these duties such as mandatory reporting for child abuse and for chemical impairment of a colleague with whom they are practicing if the colleague is not receiving treatment and is continuing to use. In these cases, the threat to the public health forms a compelling duty that overrides confidentiality. This is the case for mental health professionals who have reason to believe that a patient is a clear danger to a third party. They have a duty to break confidentiality to prevent death or harm to a third party. In most other cases where patients are posing a possible threat to others because of risky sexual practices or functioning in an impaired manner, the usual course of action is to work with the patient to mitigate risks to others.

What If My Conduct Fell Below the Standard of Care but No One Was Harmed?

Healthcare professionals cannot be liable in a negligence case—even if their conduct fell below the standard of care—if no harm resulted from their actions. There must be actual damages to a person to whom the healthcare provider owed a duty of care. However, if there is injury to a patient and all of the other elements (duty, breach, and actual and proximate cause) for negligence have been established, then a claim for professional malpractice exits.

Regardless of whether a patient is harmed, if a health professional is consistently falling below the standard of care, an issue of competency is raised. Healthcare professionals have an ethical obligation to be competent to practice. This is the rationale for mandatory continuing education and the obligation to practice free from impairment.

What if I Commit a Medical Error?

A common area of concern is medical error. It is impossible to practice for a lifetime and never commit an error. No practitioner can be 100% accurate a 100% of the time. The principle of veracity in healthcare ethics requires practitioners to be honest and forthright with information that patients have a right to. Failure to reveal mistakes and errors to patients places the practitioner at risk for litigation and malpractice charges. But just as importantly, nondisclosure erodes the bonds of trust and fidelity between patients and practitioners. Also, full and honest disclosure before the error is discovered can sometimes eliminate litigation because mitigation of the harm from the error and just compensation can be negotiated without recourse to expensive litigation. One controversial area of disclosure of errors deals with an error that has not resulted in harm to a patient. If an error is caught before the patient is harmed, then it most likely does not need to be discussed with the patient. However, the error should always be reported internally so as to investigate the process that led to the error and correct the problems to prevent further error. If the error reaches the patient and the patient has not been harmed, it is generally still recommended to discuss the error with the patient with the appropriate reassurance that no harm has occurred. If the error is not discussed and patients find out, trust will be lost even if no harm has occurred. Also, patients have a right to seek further medical consultation to make their own determination regarding potential harm of the error. Because it is their health that is at stake, they have a right to investigate the error if they choose.

The principle of veracity also applies to accurate reporting of diagnosis and procedures to insurance companies and the full disclosure of errors to companies if mistakes are made in coding and reporting.

In certain cases, medical errors may be reported to the state licensing board charged with oversight of the healthcare professional or their employer. If a healthcare professional is the accused in a board disciplinary action, they still maintain certain constitutional rights, such as (1) right of notice, (2) right of hearing, (3) right to counsel, (4) right against self-incrimination, and (5) right to judicial review. If called before a licensing board as part of any investigation or disciplinary hearing, you may want to consider speaking with an attorney to help protect your rights. Any hearing will likely be less formal than a court proceeding, but the hearing must not violate your constitutional rights, including your right to due process.

Can Employers Be Held Liable for the Conduct of the Healthcare Professionals They Employ?

The answer to this question is generally yes. There exists an accepted notion that employers have an obligation to hire and train competent employees. So employers are commonly found liable for the negligent acts of their employees. This is known as vicarious liability. An injured party has the option to file a lawsuit against both the healthcare professional and his or her employer. In many cases, only the employer is sued because the employer has greater resources. In this instance, the employer may join its employee to the litigation, but that is not required.

In litigation involving both the healthcare professional and his or her employer as defendants, it may be the case that the employer's and employee's interests are aligned and, therefore, they may share a common interest and attorney in the lawsuit. However, depending on the underlying conduct of the healthcare professional that led to the lawsuit, the employer's interests may diverge from those of the healthcare professional. It is important to remember that the same attorney cannot represent the interests of both parties when the parties' interests are not aligned. This necessities the need for the healthcare professional to hire a separate attorney to represent those interests that do not align with their employer's.

Should I Purchase Professional Liability Insurance?

Many healthcare professionals purchase professional liability insurance to insure against potential future allegations of a failure to adhere to the standard of care in the practice of their professional duties. Professional liability policies can provide for all legal costs to defend civil litigation and provide all or a portion of the money to pay any damages caused by the healthcare professional's error or malpractice. Some activities in which healthcare practitioners engage in may actually require the healthcare practitioner to maintain professional liability insurance.

What if I Witness Other Healthcare Professionals or My Employer Engaging in Unethical or Illegal Conduct?

THIS RAISES THE ISSUE OF witnessing unethical or illegal behavior at work. The healthcare professional is entrusted with the public health. Any practices, policies, and procedures that place patients at risk should be reported. Multiple state and federal laws specifically require healthcare professionals to report various types of nefarious conduct that may be witnessed in the workplace. The ethical obligations to prevent harm and do what is in the best interests of the patient compel the reporting of substandard care that can harm patients.

The normal procedure is to use the chain of command and report and document problems with health care to the responsible manager. If corrective action is not taken, then reporting to a higher level of management is warranted. In cases where an organization refuses to take action to correct harmful healthcare practices, legal action can be initiated. There are also laws in place in many states and within the federal government to protect those who report nefarious conduct. These laws are commonly referred to as whistleblower laws.

Can a Healthcare Professional Be Held Criminally Liable as a Result of a Violation Involving Professional Practice?

Criminal medical negligence is unfortunately on the rise. It is a growing trend for states to prosecute healthcare professionals for grossly negligent conduct. Some high-profile examples include conduct that involved neglecting the elderly, administering Propofol to a celebrity without proper monitoring, and dispensing contaminated epidural steroid injections, which led to 48 deaths across the country.

The difficulty is in determining the point at which, and under what standard, the healthcare professional's negligent conduct turns into a crime. Courts generally hold that to constitute a crime, there must be "gross or flagrant deviation from the standard of care" and the healthcare professional must have a "criminally culpable state of mind." Dr. James A. Filkins's (2007) research on the issues has identified the following patterns of conduct that are more likely to lead to criminal prosecution: (1) ignoring recurrences of the same problems, (2) failing to act in a timely manner, and (3) the appearance of improper motive, which involves such actions as "practicing outside of one's area of expertise" or "attempting to cover up a clinical mistake."

What Does a Typical Malpractice Case Involve?

Disputes that cannot be resolved without court intervention start when a party or parties file a complaint in court. The complaint states the facts on which the allegedly injured party or parties base their claim against the healthcare professional who allegedly injured them. After a complaint is filed, the healthcare professional must either answer the complaint by admitting or denying the complaint's allegations or move to dismiss the complaint based on its legal insufficiency.

If the complaint is not dismissed, the case moves to the discovery stage, where the parties exchange documents and information and conduct information-gathering sessions known as depositions. Almost all malpractice cases involve expert witnesses who help to define the standard of care that should be applied to the healthcare professional's alleged conduct. After fact discovery, the case may move on to trial where testimony and documents are presented to a trier of fact. The trier of fact will either be a jury of citizens or a judge. At the conclusion of the trial, the jury or the judge will render a verdict for the allegedly injured party or the healthcare professional. The losing party will then have the opportunity to appeal that verdict to a higher court.

The reality of litigating a case through trial is that it can be very burdensome, time consuming, and costly for all involved parties. As a result, the vast majority of medical malpractice cases settle prior to going to trial.

What Are Duty to Warn and Nonmaleficence?

WHETHER A HEALTHCARE PROFESSIONAL HAS a **duty to warn** a patient of a danger or risk posed by a procedure or treatment is a fundamental legal and ethical issue. From a legal perspective, courts have been reluctant to impose such a duty on anyone other than the prescribing or treating physician. The traditional basis for limiting the general duty to warn to the prescribing or treating physician is known as the learned intermediary doctrine. This doctrine is founded on the notion that the prescribing or treating physician is in the best position to determine what is best for the patient.

As such, many courts have held that other healthcare professionals do not possess a general duty to warn all patients about the risks associated with their medications. Despite the lack of a general duty to warn, however, courts have recognized many exceptions to the learned intermediary doctrine for pharmacists. Courts have been reluctant to extend these exceptions beyond pharmacists. With respect to pharmacists, the noted exceptions have become so broad that all pharmacists should, to the extent that they do not already, consider practicing as if they have a legal obligation to warn their patients of dangers or risks posed by a procedure or treatment.

By way of example, courts have held that pharmacists have a duty to warn a patient of a danger or risk posed by a medication any time (1) the pharmacist has special knowledge regarding a patient, (2) examination of the prescription shows that the patient will be harmed if the drug is used as prescribed, (3) the pharmacist voluntarily undertakes the duty, (4) the pharmacist induces the public to believe that counseling on risks of treatment will be provided, or (5) the pharmacist advertises to check for risks or dangers to the patient. Courts have been much more reluctant to create exceptions for other healthcare professionals like nurses.

From an ethical perspective, **nonmaleficence** is the ethical duty to prevent or remove harm from the patient. Because of asymmetrical knowledge, the healthcare professional has knowledge regarding the risk of medical interventions that the patient does not have. Even though patients may implicitly or explicitly consent to a medical intervention and understand the risks, the healthcare professional still has an obligation to mitigate risk by counseling the patient on concrete actions that the patient can take. For example, a pharmacist has the obligation to state the risk of a medication but also offer specific advice such as when to call the physician if a side effect appears, when to immediately stop taking the medication, or counseling on other strategies that prevent further complications from the risk.

What Are the Elements of Informed Consent and Autonomy?

INFORMED CONSENT IS GUIDED BY ethical principles, but law also recognizes it as a patient right. Providing informed consent requires healthcare providers to effectively notify patients of the (1) *nature*, (2) *risks*, (3) *benefits*, and (4) *alternatives* of a treatment or procedure. Informed consent is not obtained if the patient does not understand the presented material. At its core, informed consent is based on the patient's fundamental right to choose the best treatment in light of the information he or she has received. That fundamental right is known as **autonomy**.

Once the necessary information for informed consent is discussed with the patient, valid patient consent to the treatment or the procedure can be obtained from the patient either *expressly* (verbally or in writing) or *impliedly* (through conduct such as purchasing the medication). In emergency situations, obtaining informed consent prior to treatment may not be necessary, for example, where the patient is unconscious and therefore unable to provide consent.

Determining what information should be disclosed to the patient requires professional judgment. Failing to provide sufficient or accurate information may result in a lack of informed consent. Providing too much information may dilute the message and cause key information to get lost or unnecessarily alarm the patient regarding risk, which also may result in a lack of informed consent.

There are generally three standards of care recognized by courts to determine whether a healthcare practitioner has provided sufficient information for informed consent. Which standard of care the court will apply is largely determined by the state or federal law that the court must follow. The three general standards of care are as follows:

- **Healthcare provider–based standard:** The required disclosure of material information is based on what other reasonably prudent practitioners in the same field of practice or specialty would disclose to the patient.
- **Objective patient-based standard:** The required disclosure of material information is based on what a reasonable person would want to know about his or her treatment or procedure.
- **Subjective patient-based standard:** The required disclosure of material information is based on what the particular patient in each instance would want to know.

A healthcare practitioner's failure to obtain informed consent in accordance with the applicable standard of care may lead to liability if the patient is harmed by the treatment or the procedure.

At its most elementary level, the principle of autonomy requires that persons be treated with respect and dignity and never treated as an object. For patients to act autonomously regarding their health care they must be counseled using the principle of informed consent as the guideline. Informed consent involves counseling the patient regarding the relative risks and benefits of a proposed medical intervention and requires the following to be effective:

- Competence to understand and decide
- Freedom from undue influence or coercion
- Disclosure
- Recommendations
- Demonstration of understanding

Competency is a perquisite for both autonomy and informed consent and involves the following abilities:

- Communicate choice
- Understand consequences of choice
- Understand relevant information
- Reach a reasonable decision based on relevant risk–benefit information

A patient must first be declared incompetent based on a mental health evaluation performed by licensed mental health professionals and adjudicated by a court before the patient's autonomy can be overridden with the related obligation to informed consent. In most cases, the law does not recognize juveniles and children as autonomous until they reach the age of reason as defined by law. There are exceptions, such as the mature minor exception, that can be decided by a court.

What Constitutes an Impaired Professional?

A HEALTHCARE PROFESSIONAL IS CONSIDERED TO be an **impaired professional** when he or she (1) manifests an inability or impending inability to practice according to accepted standards as a result of substance use, abuse, or dependency or (2) is mentally or physically incompetent to carry out the duties of the profession.

Programs are available for the treatment and rehabilitation of impaired healthcare professionals. Most of these programs are designed to assist healthcare professionals with reentry into their profession. After an impaired professional is identified, a drug and alcohol assessment is conducted, treatment recommendations are made, and the impaired professional signs a treatment contract to complete the recommended treatment. Most states have an impaired professional organization composed of other recovered professionals who work with the state board in assisting with the identification and monitoring of treatment of impaired professionals.

Generally, unless a felony relating to a controlled substance is involved, punitive action is rarely taken against impaired providers. It may be possible for the impaired provider to remain in practice, provided that the impaired professional enrolls in an approved treatment plan and is regularly reporting satisfactory progress, although a medical leave may need to be granted to complete residential treatment. Impaired professional programs usually involve random drug screening to document progress.

Most states require that all healthcare providers report any professional peer or colleague when substantial evidence exists that the professional (1) has an active addictive disease for which the professional *is not receiving treatment*, (2) is diverting a controlled substance, or (3) is mentally or physically incompetent to carry out the duties of his or her profession. Any person or facility that reports in good faith and without malice is generally immune from any liability arising from such a report. On the other hand, failure to provide such a report within a reasonable time may lead to penalties, including most often a fine.

Mandatory reporting is not only a legal responsibility to protect the public health but also an ethical responsibility. Healthcare professionals who practice with impaired professionals and do not intervene become enablers, and often, the impaired practitioner draws the conclusion that managers or colleagues are not concerned or implicitly accept practice while impaired.

What Are My Licensing, Continuing Education, and Certification Obligations?

MANY HEALTHCARE PROFESSIONS REQUIRE A license to practice within a healthcare profession (e.g., dentists, nurses, osteopaths, pharmacists, physicians, physician assistants, podiatrists). Individuals who meet certain predetermined standards obtain the legal right to practice and to use a specified healthcare practitioner's title. Government boards, agencies, or departments establish licensing laws to protect the public from unqualified practitioners. These licensing bodies establish and enforce standards of practice within a profession to limit and control admission to, and practice within, the different healthcare professions.

In addition, licensing bodies often enact specific rules requiring healthcare professionals to provide proof of participation in continuing education as a prerequisite for renewal of their licenses to practice. Licensing bodies also hold the power to suspend or revoke the license of any healthcare professional who violates specific norms of conduct.

Many healthcare professionals may also seek to obtain certifications related to their scope of practice by demonstrating that their expertise meets the standards established by a particular government agency or professional group. For most healthcare professions who require a license to practice, obtaining certifications may not be mandatory.

Certification standards established by professional groups often exceed those standards of practice established for licensure by licensing bodies. In healthcare professions that do not require a license to practice, professional groups usually establish their own minimum standards for certification.

Do Gender, Race, Cultural Sensitivity, and Health Literacy Issues Apply?

VARIOUS INSTITUTIONAL, LOCAL, STATE, AND federal rules, regulations, and laws prohibit healthcare providers from discriminating on the basis of race, sex, age, religion, creed, national origin, ancestry, marital status, disability, or medical condition in providing services to their patients. Most licensed healthcare professionals and public and private healthcare business establishments that provide healthcare or medical services are prohibited from unlawfully discriminating against patients as a condition of maintaining their licenses to operate. There are numerous federal and state laws and agencies that deal with discrimination and harassment. The Equal Employment Opportunity Commission (EEOC) is a federal agency that enforces and monitors federal law, and organizations usually have a full-time EEOC office to monitor discrimination.

The principle of justice in ethics requires that all persons be treated equitably regardless of ethnic, racial, religious, or other demographic characteristics. This principle implies that for patients who cannot afford care, the practitioner has an obligation to refer or assist in finding resources through government or private agencies. Practitioners may have personal feelings or biases, but professional ethics requires that these biases are bracketed and that all persons who seek health care are treated with respect and dignity even though the practitioner may not agree with their choices.

The principle of informed consent is applicable in working with populations whose first language is not English or whose literacy skills are not sufficient to understand risk–benefit information contained in written or oral communication. It is incumbent upon the practitioner to assess health literacy because patients will not readily admit to lack of comprehension due to embarrassment or a need to not appear different. A simple request to have patients repeat back their understanding of information communicated can give an assessment of patients' level of understanding and an indication of how you must tailor communication to meet the information needs of patients. In some circumstances, interpreters may be required. It is the duty of the practitioner to ensure understanding to fulfill the requirements of informed consents.

What Are the Relevant Health Insurance Portability and Accountability Act Requirements?

THE HALLMARK OF A PROFESSIONAL is to keep information regarding a patient's health or mental health status confidential. Confidentiality in communication is an important ethical principle and has been enshrined in law by the Health Insurance Portability and Accountability Act (HIPAA) of 1996. Although the regulations in this law are extensive, there are two basic areas that healthcare practitioners need to adhere to. These are the Privacy Rule and the Security Rule. A full discussion of HIPAA is beyond the scope of this chapter. There are numerous government sources with extensive information regarding HIPAA, some of which are contained in the Suggested Readings section. The general rule of thumb for healthcare professionals should be to never reveal any information regarding a patient's treatment unless authorized by the patient or required by law. Also, healthcare professionals should make every endeavor to protect health records from being viewed by anyone with the exception of practitioners who are treating the patient and need the information for their treatment of the patient or other entities authorized by law. All healthcare practitioners who work with patients must receive HIPAA training, and all covered entities subject to the law must publically make available their compliance with HIPAA. Any entity that transmits health information is considered a covered entity. There are more extensive definitions of a covered entity available in the law.

HIPAA has regulations as to when protected health information can be disclosed and under what conditions it can be disclosed. Protected health information generally includes any treatment the patient receives such as diagnosis, diagnostic tests, prescriptions, electronic health records, counseling notes, and other information that identifies the treatment protocol of a patient. In general, protected health information cannot be disclosed without the prior authorization of the patent to whom the information belongs. In the normal course of transactions between healthcare professional and third-party payers who are responsible for payment, authorization is not needed but information should be kept to the minimum necessary to conduct the transaction.

The Security Rule establishes standards for health information communicated in electronic format. These standards include risk management, administrative safe guards, and physical and technical safeguards that protect health information from inadvertent viewing or disclosure.

What Do I Need to Know About My Employment Contract?

M OST HEALTHCARE EMPLOYERS HIRE HEALTHCARE practitioners on an "at will" basis. Employment at will means that your employment contract is for an indefinite period of time and that it may be terminated by either your employer or you at any time for any reason—good or bad—or no reason. Employment at will, however, does not mean that you are left without employee rights. A host of state and federal laws generally protect your right to fair treatment. Although states vary in the level of protection that they provide to employees, the following are a few of the many rights that state and federal laws uniformly protect:

- Right to be free from discrimination based on race, sex, age, religion, creed, national origin, ancestry, marital status, disability, or medical condition
- Right to privacy and confidentiality
- Right to be free from abuse, intimidation, and retaliatory discharge
- Right to be free from sexual harassment
- Right to refuse to participate in care
- Right to equal pay for equal work

What Obligations Come with Student Loans?

L OAN ACCEPTANCE MEANS ACCEPTING THE responsibility for repaying the money you borrow including interest costs and fees. You must repay your loans even if you do not complete your education, cannot find a job related to your professional studies, or are unhappy with your chosen profession or the education you paid for with your loan. There are only a few rare circumstances that may lead to your loans being forgiven, canceled, or discharged, such as total and permanent disability, death, and certain bankruptcy cases when undue hardship is proven.

What Are Professional Boundaries?

Professional boundaries have become of increasing importance in the modern workplace environment. Daily interaction with colleagues, sharing tasks and responsibilities, and developing long-term relationships are essential components of healthcare delivery, especially in the era of the healthcare team approach. Although it is essential to keep a distinction between personal and professional relationships in the workplace, the boundaries can be obscured at times. This can be true of relationships with both colleagues and patients.

For colleagues, specific workplaces may have policies regarding romantic or other personal relationships in the workplace. A general principle in both the law and ethics is that when a power differential exists (i.e., you have control over or can influence a person's career), a personal, romantic relationship represents a conflict of interest and must be avoided. Also when there is a blood relationship or relationship through marriage, a supervisory relationship should not exist. This poses a real or perceived conflict of interest and calls into question fairness in the workplace when one employee has a privileged relationship to a supervisor or manager.

The issue of personal and romantic relationships with patients is universally forbidden by most codes of ethics under the rubric of dual relationships. It is not permitted to have a business or romantic/sexual relationship with patients. Healthcare practitioners should also avoid such relationships with a patient's spouse. The power differential and dynamics of a healthcare provider–patient relationship place the patient at a disadvantage, and therefore, this situation is rife for the possibility of exploitation. The following characteristics will assist in differentiating a professional and personal relationship and can be used as criteria for deciding when professional and personal boundaries are becoming blurred.

Professional Relationships

- There is money exchanged for service.
- Relationship is limited to a specific intervention.
- Service is in a professional setting.
- The relationships are defined by the service provided.
- Sharing of personal information is one -way from patient to provider.

- The provider establishes and maintains the relationship within the guidelines of professional standards and ethics.
- The relationship is based on the particular competency and expertise of the professional.
- The relationship exists for the benefit of the patient, not the provider.

Personal Relationships

- Money may not be involved or shared.
- The relationship is not limited by a service.
- The rules of the relationship are mutually agreed upon.
- The relationship tends to be unstructured.
- Power is shared and negotiated.
- The relationship is mutually established and maintained.
- No special training is required.
- Mutual satisfaction and benefit are the basis.

Conclusion

THE LEGAL AND ETHICAL ASPECTS of healthcare professionalism require an altruistic motive. Protecting patients from reasonably foreseeable harm, striving to do what is in the best interests of patients, and ensuring equitable treatment of all patients regardless of personal or social characteristics form the basis of professional duties. In addition, respecting patient privacy, ensuring both personal and organizational integrity in the delivery of health care, and being forthright and honest with patients, colleagues, regulators, and insurance companies support these obligations. Maintaining competency through continuing education and study and ensuring that professionals do not practice impaired are obligations to protect the public. These obligations, coupled with understanding and maintaining professional boundaries in the workplace with both patients and colleagues, will support professional environments that place patient well-being as the goal of all healthcare practices.

What Do the Practitioners/Others Say?

FOR NEXT CLASS, BE PREPARED to discuss the legal and ethical aspects of practice based on any *one* of the following:

- A discussion with your colleagues, or others, on how they feel and what they know about legal and ethical issues in practice.
- An article on a legal or ethical issue of practice either from the research literature or any other source.
- A movie, television program, or YouTube video about the legal and ethical issues in practice.
- A book on legal and ethical issues in practice (literary, historical, psychological, or any other source).

The Students: Personal and Professional Issues

B ASED ON THE DESCRIPTION OF each student at the beginning of the chapter, what are the personal and professional issues (either immediately or in the future) confronting each student? Consider whether they are linked and, if so, how. Finally, what would you recommend to each student to resolve these issues?

Dana S.

Personal Issues

Professional Issues

Are They Linked? Will the Personal Issues Impact Professional Behavior?

Recommendations

Ivan T.

Personal Issues

Professional Issues

Are They Linked? Will the Personal Issues Impact Professional Behavior?

Recommendations

Niki M.

Personal Issues

Professional Issues

Are They Linked? Will the Personal Issues Impact Professional Behavior?

Recommendations

Ryan P.

Personal Issues

Professional Issues

Are They Linked? Will the Personal Issues Impact Professional Behavior?

Recommendations

Exercises

1. With several of your classmates, review the board structure and membership in your state. Review the kinds of issues the board takes action on and the penalties meted out.

2. If a colleague at work asks you to "bend" the rules for him or her, should you do it? How far should you go? Which rules, if any, should you bend?

3. If a patient asks you to "bend" the rules for him or her, should you do it? How far should you go? Which rules, if any, should you bend?

4. Write a one-page executive summary of the chapter.

5. Review the mind map from the opening of the chapter. Would you change anything following reading the chapter?

Case Example

Eighty-one-year-old Jack Horn was prescribed Coumadin, a blood thinner, by his physician assistant, Jennifer, in a dosage of 10 mg on the first day and then 5 mg per day thereafter. Jennifer's office called in the prescription via telephone to the pharmacy. The oral prescription order was taken by a pharmacist, Sherri, who correctly transcribed the prescription and then left for the day, leaving another pharmacist, Arnold, to fill the prescription.

Arnold filled the prescription with the correct medication, warfarin (a generic form of Coumadin), but the instructions set forth on the bottle label instructed Mr. Horn to "TAKE TWO [5 MG] TABLETS BY MOUTH EVERY DAY THEN TAKE 1 TABLET IN THE EVENING," a dosage that was three times the dosage prescribed. Mr. Horn's visiting nurse, Joe, administered the medication to Mr. Horn in accordance with the instructions set forth on the label of the bottle. Shortly after, Mr. Horn suffered a stroke that resulted in permanent injuries.

Mr. Horn sued Jennifer (his physician assistant), the pharmacy, Sherri and Arnold (his pharmacists), and Joe (his nurse). In connection with this lawsuit, Arnold was deposed and testified that he had an obligation to learn information about the medications that he was dispensing, such as the dosage. He stated that he had to know the recommended dosages "so that we can be aware of excess dosages that could cause harm." He also testified that he knew that Coumadin was a "High Therapeutic Index" medication, meaning a medication where even a small dosage error can cause serious health consequences to a patient. He further admitted that he did not know the safe loading dose, and he was aware that this lack of knowledge placed a patient at serious risk.

At the time of the incident, the pharmacy's computer system contained a program called the "Gold Standard," which contained information about all prescription medications, including the medications' recommended dosages, potential allergic reactions, and medication contraindications. It also contained information about the patients, including the patients' disease states, other medications that had been and were being taken by the patient, and the patients' drug allergies. If the prescribed dosage exceeded the recommended daily dosage, then the computer would display a yellow flag and would instruct the pharmacist to "verify the dosage." The computer in this case displayed a yellow warning to Arnold, and he admitted receiving the warning and that he was required to contact the prescribing physician to verify the dosage. Instead of contacting the physician, he overrode the warning and dispensed the medication.

Joe was also deposed, and he testified that he thought the dose was high based on his 5 years of experience and several years of schooling. He also testified that he called Jennifer's office to question the dosage, but that the individual who answered the phone confirmed that she phoned the prescription into the pharmacy correctly. Joe admitted that he thought the medication could injure Mr. Horn, but that ultimately he "trusted that the pharmacists and the physician assistant knew what they were doing." Joe admitted that he did not contact either the pharmacy or the prescribing physician assistant.

1. Who do you think could be potentially liable to Mr. Horn? Why?

2. What defines the standard of care of these healthcare professionals?

3. Does Arnold's conduct constitute criminal medical negligence?

4. What ethical obligations are in play for these healthcare professionals?

5. What types of medication errors occur in healthcare settings, and what is the obligation to inform patients of errors? Is it ever justified to withhold information?

6. What is the incidence of medication errors in healthcare?

7. What role do work load and work conditions play in medication errors?

8. What types of information should be disclosed when a medication error occurs?

9. If errors are minor and caught early before there is any harm, should they be disclosed to patients?

What's Important to You in the Chapter?

WITH SEVERAL OF YOUR CLASSMATES, discuss the idea or ideas most likely to effect a change in your values, attitudes, or behaviors. Be succinct. Write no more than two sentences.

Reference

Filkins, J. A. (2007). *Criminalization of Medical Negligence: Legal Medicine* (7th ed.). Philadelphia, PA: Elsevier.

Suggested Readings

Abood, R. (2005). *Pharmacy Practice and Law* (4th ed.). Sudbury, MA: Jones and Bartlett Publishers.

Beauchum, P., and Childross, J. F. (2012). *Principles of Biomedical Ethics*. New York: Oxford University Press.

Gillon, R. (1994). Medical ethics: Four principles plus attention to scope. *British Medical Journal*. 309 (6948), 184–189.

Guido, G. W. (2009). *Legal & Ethical Issues in Nursing* (6th ed.). Upper Saddle River, NJ: Prentice Hall.

Hall, M. A., Bobinski, M. A., and Orentlicher, D. (2013). *Health Care Law and Ethics* (8th ed.). New York: Aspen Publishers.

Hall, M. A., and Ellman, I. M. (2011). *Health Care law and Ethics in a Nutshell* (3rd ed.). St. Paul, MN: West Publishing.

Macklin, R. (2003). Applying the four principles. *Journal of Medical Ethics*. 29 (5), 275–280.

Pozgar, G. D. (2013). *Legal and Ethical Issues for Health Professionals* (3rd ed.). Burlington, MA: Jones & Bartlett Learning.

U.S. Department of Health and Human Services. (2015). Understanding health information privacy. www.hhs.gov/ocr/privacy/hipaa/understanding. Accessed August 6, 2015.

Veatch, R. M., Haddad, A. M., and English, D. C. (2010). *Case Studies in Biomedical Ethics*. New York: Oxford University Press.

Veatch, R. M., and Harley, F. (1997). *Case Studies in Allied Health Ethics*. Upper Saddle River, NJ: Prentice Hall.

Glossary

Academic dishonesty taking a cognitive shortcut

Academic entitlement the idea that a student deserves a grade or special treatment regardless of input

Academic incivility anything that disrupts the classroom

Accountability being responsible for one's actions

Agreeableness the personality trait of being cooperative, trusting, and empathic

Altruism willingness to serve the best interest of the patient rather than your self-interest

Analytical thinking thinking that is deliberate and conscious

Autonomy the patient's right to choose

Burnout the loss of energy, idealism, and purpose due to stress and work

Collaborative professional relationships mutual power, trust, and respect

Collegial professional relationships equal power, trust, and respect

Compassion fatigue the exhaustion that overtakes a person that causes a decline in their ability to function as a result of helping others

Conscientiousness the personality trait of being disciplined, organized, goal driven, and self-controlled

Consummate professional focuses on the patient and the job

Credibility being trusted and believed in

Culture the way things are done at work; the collective beliefs, values, principles, norms, symbols, systems, and habits that guide work behavior

Deliberate practice a well-defined task, appropriate level of difficulty, informed feedback, and repetition and correction

Duty commitment to serve the patient

Duty to warn obligation of healthcare provider to patient to provide information

Emotional labor the requirement of the job to display certain emotions

Emotions a feeling and its distinctive thoughts, psychological and biological states, and range of propensities to act

Ethics what one ought or ought not to do

Excellence conscientious commitment to improvement

Exemplification letting others know how hard you work

Experiential learning the four-stage process by which people learn from their experiences

Expertise up-to-date knowledge, highly developed perceptual abilities, a sense of what is relevant, an ability to simplify complex problems, an ability to adapt to exceptions, and ability to perceive meaningful patterns in large amounts of data

Extraversion the personality trait of focusing outward, liking action more than reflection, and enjoying other people's company

Friendly stranger professional relationships little trust and acknowledgement; courteous and formal

Generational theory people of approximately the same age exhibit similar attitudes, behaviors, and beliefs

Honor and integrity commitment to the highest standards of behavior

Hostile, adversarial, and abusive professional relationships negative in tone and action

Impaired professional a practitioner incapable of performing his or her duties due to mental or physical causes

Implementing professional choices the ability to carry out professional choices

Informed consent notifying patients of the consequences of their treatment

Ingratiation taking an interest in others' personal lives

Intimidation letting others know you will not be pushed around

Intuition thinking that is unconscious and rapid

Judgment the ability to infer, estimate, and predict the character of unknown events; what you use if you do not have enough information

Law a body of rules, standards, and principles used to govern conduct

Liability who is responsible in a legal sense

Machiavellianism valuing expedience over principle, manipulative tactics for personal gain, and a cynical view of human nature

Millennial those born between 1980 and 2000

Mindset a belief that impacts behavior

Moral outrages healthcare workers who deliberately harm patients

Narcissism an inflated view of self and fantasies of control, admiration, and success

Negligence a deficiency in care

Neuroticism the personality trait of being anxious, insecure, and prone to stress and worry

Nonmaleficence do no harm

Openness to experience the personality trait of being creative, imaginative, and preferring variety over routine

Personal and professional growth change in a positive direction

Personality the enduring pattern of thoughts, feelings, and behaviors that distinguish individuals from another

Practical intelligence knowing how to get things done

Professional judgment identifying and selecting courses of action

Professional motivation the priority an individual assigns to professional obligations

Professional sensitivity perception and interpretation of situations requiring a professional response

Professionalism guiding beliefs and ideals based on a commitment to standards of excellence in practice, a commitment to the interest of the patient, and a commitment to the needs of the community

Professor/boss focuses on being right, whether or not that is the case

Prudent paranoia prudent suspicion at work that something is happening that will affect you

Psychological capital an individual's positive psychological state of development that negates the debilitating aspects of work

Psychological contract a person's beliefs about the terms of an exchange

Psychopathy a lack of concern for others and the rules of society coupled with likeability, glibness, and charm

Relationship management the balance between doing things to preserve the relationship and preserving personal integrity

Resilience the ability to respond to acute and chronic stress

Respect for others belief in the value of all human beings

Schema mental blueprints and theories of the world

Self-awareness the ability to understand who you are

Self-directed learning identifying personal learning needs, determining the learning objective, deciding how to evaluate outcomes, and identifying learning strategies

Self-efficacy the belief that one can cope with and accomplish difficult tasks

Self-management behaving appropriate to the context

Self-promotion letting others know of your talents and qualifications

Social awareness paying attention to the people and the world around you

Strategic thinking a cold, hard, analytical looks at trends, statistics, and graphs unfettered by emotions to understand the future

Student consumerism the view that college is just another consumer marketplace and a university education is just another product

Student/employee focuses on learning or negatively shirking responsibility

Student—teacher professional relationships both parties are willing to listen, teach, and learn

Stupidity not thinking, or thinking becoming frozen

Supplication trying to gain sympathy so others will help you

Tacit knowledge knowledge of how the world works gained from experience

Toxic political environment a workplace that is at war and where everyone is out for themselves

Wisdom expertise in the fundamentals of life; knowing what is important in life

Worry the cognitive component of anxiety

Index

Note: "Page numbers followed by *b* and *f* indicate material in boxes and figures, respectively."